11/1/18
$22.95
AS-14
11/18

Vaccines Did Not Cause Rachel's Autism

Other Books by Peter J. Hotez

Forgotten People, Forgotten Diseases:
The Neglected Tropical Diseases and Their Impact
on Global Health and Development

Blue Marble Health: An Innovative Plan to
Fight Diseases of the Poor amid Wealth

Vaccines Did Not Cause Rachel's Autism

MY JOURNEY AS A VACCINE SCIENTIST, PEDIATRICIAN, AND AUTISM DAD

Peter J. Hotez, MD, PhD

Foreword by Arthur L. Caplan
Division of Medical Ethics
NYU School of Medicine

Johns Hopkins University Press
Baltimore

© 2018 Johns Hopkins University Press
All rights reserved. Published 2018
Printed in the United States of America on acid-free paper
2 4 6 8 9 7 5 3 1

Johns Hopkins University Press
2715 North Charles Street
Baltimore, Maryland 21218-4363
www.press.jhu.edu

Library of Congress Cataloging-in-Publication Data

Names: Hotez, Peter J., author.
Title: Vaccines did not cause Rachel's autism: My journey as a vaccine scientist, pediatrician, and autism dad / Peter J. Hotez ; Foreword by Arthur L. Caplan.
Description: Baltimore, Maryland : Johns Hopkins University Press, [2018] | Includes bibliographical references and index.
Identifiers: LCCN 2018002311 | ISBN 9781421426600 (hc. : alk. paper) | ISBN 9781421426617 (electronic) | ISBN 1421426609 (hc. : alk. paper) | ISBN 1421426617 (electronic)
Subjects: | MESH: Vaccination—trends | Vaccines | Autism Spectrum Disorder—etiology | Health Knowledge, Attitudes, Practice | Science | Anti-Vaccination Movement | Health Communication
Classification: LCC RJ240 | NLM WA 115 | DDC 614.4/7083—dc23
LC record available at https://lccn.loc.gov/2018002311

A catalog record for this book is available from the British Library.

Special discounts are available for bulk purchases of this book. For more information, please contact Special Sales at 410-516-6936 or specialsales@press.jhu.edu.

Johns Hopkins University Press uses environmentally friendly book materials, including recycled text paper that is composed of at least 30 percent post-consumer waste, whenever possible.

To my amazing wife of 30 years, Ann Elizabeth Hotez, the most brilliant and devoted mother of four adult children.

To Rachel, to whom I am grateful for her incredible enthusiasm in participating in this book. I thank her for our detailed discussions on autism and vaccines during weekly walks in the neighborhood.

I want to express my family's deep appreciation to the joyful inhabitants, friends, merchants, and service workers of Montrose, Houston, who daily show love and kindness to Rachel.

Finally, I want to say thank you to my public health heroes at the Houston Health Department; Harris County Public Health and Environmental Services; Texas Department of State Health Services; US Centers for Disease Control and Prevention; National Institute of Allergy and Infectious Diseases; Fogarty International Center; US National Institutes of Health; US Public Health Service; Walter Reed Army Institute of Research in the Department of Defense; United Nations Children's Fund; World Health Organization; World International Property Organization; Coalition for Epidemic Preparedness Innovations; Gavi, the Vaccine Alliance; Carlos Slim Foundation; Kleberg Foundation; Southwest Electronic Energy Medical Research Institute; Blavatnik Charitable Foundation; European Union; Japanese Global Health Innovative Technology Fund; Brockman Medical Research Foundation; Bill & Melinda Gates Foundation; and, of course, Baylor College of Medicine and Texas Children's Hospital. Thanks go also to the Mort and Chris Hyman family, to Bill and Melinda Kacal, and to Rebecca Marvil and Brian Smyth.

Contents

Foreword

Why is this book needed? And why must I urge you to read it? Isn't the case for vaccination already clear?

Most of us do seem to know that vaccines work and that they are safe. Most Americans get their kids vaccinated. Pediatricians, among the most trusted doctors there are, firmly believe in them. People around the world are eager to prevent polio, cholera, rotavirus disease, cervical cancer, and measles from disabling or killing them by using vaccines. And don't we all dream of the day when HIV, malaria, herpes, and other horrible infectious diseases could meet the same fate as smallpox—gone from our planet thanks to vaccination?

Yet, despite the fact that vaccination is among the most important and effective interventions medicine has ever discovered, doubts and fears about the practice still exist. You may trust in vaccination, but you probably know someone who doesn't. Public support for vaccination is still somewhat frail in many parts of the world. Some of the best-educated people in this and other nations harbor reservations about vaccine safety. And organized political resistance to vaccination continues to rear its dangerous head in many communities.

Why is this so? The reasons for doubts and fears about vaccines are complicated.

Vaccination is, relatively speaking, new. The conquest of polio, a key triumph of vaccination, took place in the 1950s and 1960s. New things still breed distrust. And vaccine success has been so amazing—with many families in the developed world never encountering a case of tetanus, polio, measles, meningitis, or diphtheria—that any risk from vaccination, no matter how tiny, seems intolerable. Vaccines have worked so well that they lull us into a false confidence that the plagues of our grandparents and great-grandparents are simply gone forever. And who needs to vaccinate when there are other "options" such as essential oils, tea, neti pots, blueberry massage, energy therapy, chiropractic treatment, and vitamins to stave off the flu and other contagious diseases? These useless nostrums have plenty of advocates who don't seem to hear the viruses and bacteria laughing at them.

False claims about vaccine safety have gotten into social media where, like vampires, they live on in the darkest parts of the Internet forever. Vaccines are tied up with other issues and institutions that produce strong negative feelings, like Big Pharma and government restrictions on personal liberty. And perhaps most important, until this book, proponents of vaccines have made their case mainly with abstract statistics. Critics pay little attention to numbers. Rightly or wrongly, they invoke identifiable individuals, almost always kids, almost always their child, to justify their concerns about vaccine safety.

My friend Dr. Peter Hotez is the world's leading authority on battling tropical diseases. Worried about Zika, Ebola, West Nile virus, typhus, malaria—he is your man. He is a pediatrician who also knows one heck of a lot about vaccines. He has also thought long and hard about vaccine safety. He has tangled with the disgraced former British doctor Andrew Wakefield, who promulgated a false causal link between vaccines and autism that led to many preventable cases of measles and other diseases as parents ducked what they were told was the reason for autism. Wakefield now lives in Texas where Hotez, from his office in Houston, keeps an eye on his ongoing anti-vaccine craziness and moneymaking "cures." Hotez does this while bearing the price of his vigilance in the form of threatening, hateful e-mails and tweets from Wakefield's supporters, who like Japanese soldiers on remote Pacific islands who fought on long after World War II had ended with Japan's defeat, keep up the vaccine-autism myth despite a mountain of evidence to the contrary.

Why might vaccine safety in general and the claim that vaccines cause autism concern Peter Hotez? Well, there is the professional, academic desire to set the factual record straight. But there is another, deeply personal reason: Peter Hotez and his wife, Ann, have an autistic daughter, Rachel. Obviously, the Hotez family wants to know why Rachel has a disability. And when anti-vaccinators impugn vaccines as the cause of autism, they all pay close attention. A man who has spent his career fighting neglected tropical diseases, sometimes with vaccines, is going to be especially and appropriately concerned when vaccines are flagged over and over again as the cause of his own daughter's health issues.

Hotez introduces you to Rachel and Ann and the rest of his family in the book. He tells you about his life with an autistic baby, child, and adult. He does, as he should, let Rachel speak her mind about her autism. And he shows you, as no scientist or vaccine expert has ever done before, why it is not true that

Rachel is autistic because of vaccines. He proves to you that current science shows that no child is autistic as a result of vaccination—it is simply impossible.

Dogged anti-vaccinators will hate this book. Not only does the author know the science from firsthand experience, experience that the critics lack, he knows as well as anyone the challenge and the rewards that an autistic child brings to a dad and a family. If anyone were to have a reason to buy into the lie that is the vaccine-autism connection, it would be Peter Hotez. While he is willing to pursue the truth anywhere it leads, as any good scientist must, he understands that science finds the roots of autism nowhere near visits to the pediatrician to get the vaccines that prevent the many diseases that can and, sadly for some, still do maim and kill our children.

When an erudite, highly trained scientist who is a true hero for his work in saving the world's poor and downtrodden shares his knowledge and clinical insights along with his parental experience, when his beliefs in the value of what he does are put to the test of a life guiding his own child's challenges, then you must pay attention. You should. This book brings to an end the link between autism and vaccination. Not because Peter and Rachel and Ann have lived with autism but because autism has been the forge that has made Peter articulate an impregnable argument that vaccines do not cause autism. You can hardly ask more of an author and a book on vaccines and autism than that.

Arthur L. Caplan

Drs. William F. and Virginia Connolly Mitty Professor of Bioethics,
Department of Population Health
Director, Division of Medical Ethics

NYU School of Medicine

Preface

While my previous books have certainly contained self-reflections, this one makes a deeply personal statement as both a vaccine scientist and the father of an adult daughter with autism. Its major audience includes scientists, university students, pediatricians and their patients, and all parents or guardians who have heard bad or unsavory things about vaccines. The book provides an alternative and scientifically sound counter-narrative to an aggressive and growing national and international anti-vaccine movement. The book spells out why vaccines are both safe and extraordinary lifesaving technologies. It highlights evidence that vaccines do not cause autism, but it also takes the reader through one additional step by explaining what we now know about the modern neurobiology of autism. It explains an absence of a plausible link between vaccines and autism, and why vaccines could not possibly be responsible for the autism spectrum disorder.

I wrote this book now because the anti-vaccine, or anti-vaxxer, movement has grown so strong and powerful. As of this writing, a terrible measles outbreak is finally winding down in Minnesota, with many children hospitalized. The 2017 Minnesota epidemic follows on the heels of an equally large and serious one in California. Furthermore, tens of thousands of parents have chosen to exempt their kids from vaccinations in the state of Texas (for nonmedical reasons)—to the point where I believe that measles outbreaks there are inevitable. Currently, 18 US states allow nonmedical exemptions for reasons of personal or philosophical beliefs, and some major metropolitan areas, including Seattle and Phoenix, are also at imminent risk of measles outbreaks. Because these actions have been met largely with silence from US government agencies, the American anti-vaccine movement is proceeding mostly unopposed. I do not mean this as a political statement that favors one political party or another. The fact is that Washington, DC, has generally not attempted to counteract anti-vaccine activities since they resurged in the early 2000s. The silence has continued through various presidential administrations.

The situation may even be worse across the Atlantic Ocean. In Romania and elsewhere in Europe, we are seeing an unprecedented return of measles cases and outbreaks. Anti-vaccine sentiments are now pervasive in countries such as France and Croatia. And now there is the risk that we could see measles yet again in the large low- and middle-income countries of Brazil, Russia, India, Indonesia, China, and Nigeria. A return of measles and other childhood infections to these nations would reverse child mortality figures, which have been trending downward since the creation of the United Nations Millennium Development Goals in 2000. This would be a catastrophe.

Today, measles ranks among the most deadly of childhood infections, yet parents and guardians are walking away from protecting their children against this and other deadly scourges in unprecedented numbers. They are abandoning the option of protecting their children because of phony propaganda released by an anti-vaccine movement that began in

1998. Since then, the movement has become scary, powerful, and well organized. One aspiration of this book is to counter the claims of the anti-vaccine movement that MMR (measles-mumps-rubella) and other childhood vaccines are either unsafe or cause autism. By providing a personal account as a vaccine researcher and father of an autistic child, I hope to explain in a straightforward manner why their assertions are false.

Several excellent and detailed accounts have been published previously about the rise of the anti-vaccine movement, especially in the United States. They include excellent accounts written by Paul Offit and Seth Mnookin. My book does not attempt to revisit those topics. Instead, it is intended as a highly concise summary of why vaccines are safe and cannot possibly cause autism, as the anti-vaccine lobby asserts. The book also highlights the steps by which the biological sequence of events leading to autism evolve—beginning during pregnancy. It explains why some parents might mistakenly believe vaccines could cause autism, a misunderstanding that the anti-vaccine groups effectively exploit.

To make this book effective, I believed I had to reveal a fair bit of personal information about myself, my family, and especially Rachel, who as of this writing is a 25-year-old adult with autism spectrum disorder. In my discussions with her—as well as in her conversations with my wife, Ann—Rachel has been excited to be featured in the book. She is eager to tell her story and thinks that it represents a way in which she can make an important contribution. But for our family, this book is definitely out of our comfort zone. It was not easy putting so much out there about Rachel and ourselves. In doing so, I took as many precautions as possible to protect or shield them from potential critics and avoided revealing details that might be considered too intimate or even exploitative. However, on a number of occasions, I had some serious doubts about whether going into specifics about Rachel's autism was appropriate, but I felt encouraged by Rachel's enthusiasm, her eagerness to tell the story, and the potential benefits of a straightforward account of autism spectrum disorder, together with an in-depth analysis of why this condition is not linked to vaccines. In the end, I am hopeful this book will reap public health benefits.

I want to thank Ann for preserving all of Rachel's school records and other documents, making it possible for me to retrace her history. I also want to thank Nathaniel Wolf (yet again) for his editorial assistance with this book, Robin Coleman at Johns Hopkins University Press for championing my ideas, and Vernesta Jackson for her assistance. I especially want to thank Mojie Crigler, my editor who provided so many helpful suggestions, especially for her advice on how to better illustrate Rachel's true character and amplify Ann's voice. She also provided great advice on how to reorder my narrative to create a more compelling story. I also want to thank Laura Biel from *Texas Monthly* magazine, who made a great effort to tell the story about vaccines and autism and our life with Rachel in a feature article in December 2017, and also the amazing photographer for that piece, Brian Goldman. One of Brian's images is included in this book. I also want to express my appreciation to Arthur Caplan at New York University for agreeing to write the cogent foreword.

Another strong impetus for writing this book is what I perceive to be a dearth of voices speaking out against the modern anti-vaccine movement. Their false claims and public statements more often than not go unchallenged. I hope that this book might serve as a clarion call for other scientists and physicians to speak out on behalf of science. For too long, scientists have been discouraged from engaging the public. Through a new initiative, which I term "science tikkun," I hope to reverse this long-standing but ultimately detrimental practice.

Finally, I want to thank my mentors and colleagues at Baylor College of Medicine (especially Baylor president, Paul Klotman), Texas Children's Hospital (especially Texas Children's CEO, Mark Wallace, and physician-in-chief, Mark Kline), Baylor University, Texas A&M University, and the James A. Baker III Institute for Public Policy at Rice University (especially Ambassador Edward Djerejian and Françoise Djerejian) for their unwavering support and encouragement. I also want to express my gratitude for the support of my friends and colleagues at the National School of Tropical Medicine at Baylor College of Medicine and the incredibly dedicated scientists of the Texas Children's Center for Vaccine Development, a unique nonprofit product development partnership making vaccines against the world's neglected diseases. Our scientists are my inspiration.

· 1 ·

Family Interrupted

On the sort of warm and clear afternoon when you finally realize that winter is actually done, I drove home from the Yale University School of Medicine. My work, leading a biomedical research laboratory devoted to making the first vaccine for human hookworm infection, was exciting but demanding and usually required me to work on weekends. That Saturday I pulled into the driveway to find my wife, Ann, standing in front of our house with our two oldest children, Matt and Emy, who were then nine and seven years old, respectively. No one looked happy, and Ann looked tired. Our five-year-old daughter Rachel had disappeared—again—and no one could find her. "I don't think she went far; I just had my back turned for a few minutes," Ann explained. "So I can't figure out where she went this time."

Almost three years before, Rachel had been diagnosed as having pervasive developmental disorder–not otherwise specified (PDD-NOS), an outdated term for what is now called autism spectrum disorder (ASD). Taking flight was a prominent feature of Rachel's PDD-NOS. She loved the sensation of running and would usually laugh while fleeing. I'm not sure what it was about running that gave Rachel satisfaction, although I recognize that wandering off is not uncommon for kids with ASD. In Rachel's case, we often felt that part of the excitement was getting a reaction from us as we gave chase and retrieved her.

When Rachel ran off, she could cover a lot of distance, fast, and she wouldn't respond to our shouts and pleas to return. Often she would wind up in different parts of our neighborhood. If we saw her take off, we dropped everything and chased her. Someone from the Hotez family running after Rachel was a common sight in our neighborhood, and often a caring neighbor would join in. Saturday morning soccer games were a special nightmare. Both Matt and Emy played soccer, but oftentimes neither Ann nor I could sit with the other parents and actually watch the games. Rather than enjoying Matt's and Emy's competitions like the other parents, we were instead consumed with running after a laughing Rachel with her red curls flying as she sped across all of the playing fields. Like many of our family experiences, soccer would sometimes become an exhausting and dreary endeavor.

Cheshire, Connecticut, was an idyllic New England town with good schools, playgrounds with beautifully crafted swing sets, quaint pizza and ice cream parlors, an ice hockey rink where our son Matt played, pretty leaves in the fall, and a hill for sledding in the winter. Our neighborhood was full of families, almost all of whom knew Rachel. However, if Rachel ran out of our immediate vicinity, it became especially awkward for Ann, and she often felt judged or embarrassed. Once we caught her, we would have to physically restrain her. Sometimes she would then try to run away again. An otherwise quiet, pleasant afternoon in lovely Cheshire would turn into a frantic, panicked, stressful search-and-rescue mission.

Running was just one of Rachel's impulsive behaviors. She

was also fascinated with throwing objects or dumping things onto the floor or into the toilet. Our house sometimes resembled the aftermath of an earthquake at Toys R Us. Whatever Rachel held in her hands had to be tossed: food, toys, or her new Stride Rite sneakers, which she dropped out of the car window onto the Merritt Parkway at 60 mph. Rachel's autism is not the type of autism that is typically featured in the press or well described to the public. First, Rachel is a girl, whereas boys constitute the majority of people with ASD. Second, Rachel is highly verbal and interactive (often in odd, sometimes destructive ways), in contrast to many on the spectrum, especially boys.

Her adventures often got us into difficult or even scary situations. Rachel's flights meant it was nearly impossible to take family vacations or have even modest outings as a family. Her autism demanded all hands on deck, including her siblings'. On this particular Saturday, Ann and the kids first went into the woods behind our house to hunt for Rachel, and then we piled in the car and drove to Rachel's usual spots, such as a local playground. Nothing. Back home, we started phoning neighbors. Had anyone seen her run by? No. Across the street lived a teenager named Kevin and his mother, Barbara. When I called their number, Rachel answered.

"Rachel, what are you doing in Kevin's home?" I asked.

"I'm looking in their refrigerator and at their photo album," she replied.

"Rachel, get Kevin and put him on the phone."

"Kevin's not here."

"Well, then get me Barbara."

"Barbara's not here either." There was excitement in her voice.

"Rachel, who is in the house with you?

"Nobody's home, just me."

She had crawled through the pet entrance to enjoy an afternoon of Kevin and Barbara's hospitality by herself. Unable to reach Kevin or Barbara, we turned to Matt, who could still barely fit through the pet entrance. With an angry look, he went in and retrieved Rachel, telling us afterward to never again make a similar request!

With everyone back home, we called the Cheshire police department in case Rachel had broken or disturbed anything in the house. She was, in a sense, breaking and entering, and although she didn't see it that way, we wanted to give her a clear message that this behavior was unacceptable. A police cruiser came to the house. The officer's major concern was whether anything was taken from the house or damaged, and whether the property owner—Barbara—cared or wanted to press charges. Barbara was gracious, and it helped that she herself was a special needs teacher's aide in Rachel's school. Rachel had a flat response to the arrival of the Cheshire police. It didn't seem to register with her. The policeman spoke to Rachel, but all she could articulate was that she "wanted to see Barbara's pictures." Rachel showed no real remorse and also no embarrassment. She seemed to have no sense or understanding that what she did might have put her in danger.

Afterward we tried our best to give Matt and Emy a calm ending to their Saturday, taking them out for pizza, and then having them spend time with their friends. For Ann these types of stressful experiences with Rachel had become a new normal, and Ann did her best to continue her daily activities. Inwardly, however, the constant stress of having a daughter with ASD, especially one so physically and emotionally demanding, became a source of great sadness, ultimately leading to clinical depression that required both pharmacologic treatment and talk therapy. My sadness mostly remained hidden or known only to Ann. I was determined not to let chaotic family conditions interfere with my deep connection to our other children or my dream of becoming a scientist.

My Start in Science

My own childhood was quiet, nurturing, and marked by an early fascination with science, maps, and exotic places. Like so many who went into microbiology, I was enormously affected by Paul de Kruif's *Microbe Hunters,* a paperback compendium of the lives of the great microbiologists, such as Louis Pasteur, Robert Koch, and Walter Reed. I was fascinated by how these individuals went about making discoveries and the challenges they faced from their scientific peers or a skeptical public. I was impressed by their resilience in the face of hardships, which ultimately became very good life lessons.

I was born in Hartford, Connecticut, and then my solidly middle-class family moved to West Hartford. Although neither of my parents were scientists, I had some important family role models. My maternal uncle, Irv Goldberg, is a Harvard biochemist and cancer pharmacologist, now retired in his 90s, and my mother's uncle, David Krech, was a University of California at Berkeley psychologist (and social activist), who was once appointed by Judge Thurgood Marshall to provide expert testimony on the harmful effects of segregation. We lived near a small brook from which I would sample stagnant water, bringing it back to a small laboratory that I had initially set up in my upstairs bedroom, but because of the occasional spill or mess and funny smells—and at my parents' request—was relocated to our basement.

A good part of my youth was spent peering through a

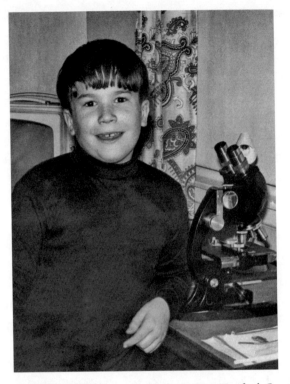

FIGURE 1. "Living large" with my microscope in West Hartford, Connecticut, circa 1960s

microscope at all sorts of protozoa and rotifers (fig. 1). At my side always was a worn paperback copy of Johnson and Bleifeld's 1963 book, *Hunting with a Microscope*. What I remember most was that the book was filled with lots of interesting diagrams of microorganisms—animals and plants that I had never dreamed existed. The pictures inspired me to want to see these life forms firsthand. Whatever I couldn't find in our local brook or roadside puddles, I used my allowance—$1 a week from my grandfather, Morris Goldberg—to save up and buy mail-order specimens from the Carolina Biological Supply Company. Back then, via the US Parcel Post, living organisms in water would be sent to our home in small transparent jars with white screw-top covers. I would use an eyedropper to pick up what was inside, place it on a glass slide, and then apply the cover slip. An entire new world opened up, one that I found incredibly exciting. Later, while I was in high school, I was privileged to work at the nearby University of Connecticut School of Medicine in the laboratory of Dr. Bob Poyton, studying yeast and exploring the newly developing science of molecular biology.

Another fascination of mine at that time (and to some extent still today) was maps and geographic atlases. I loved learning about distant places, and my favorite *Microbe Hunters* stories were the ones that took place in Africa, Asia, and Latin America. Looking back, I think it was the fascination with microorganisms and maps that early on prompted me to combine these two interests when deciding on a career path. By the time I entered college, I knew that I was going to study parasitic and tropical diseases in faraway locales. At Yale University, where an outstanding group of investigators were studying parasitic organisms, I did lots of undergraduate research in the laboratories of Professor Curtis Patton, and later Professor Frank Richards, who took me under his wing.

Curtis Patton was one of the first African American full professors at Yale University School of Medicine. After attending Fisk University and Michigan State University, Curtis had studied parasitology at Rockefeller University under the legendary William Trager (1910–2005), the first scientist to successfully cultivate malaria in the laboratory. Afterward, Curtis set up his own Yale laboratory devoted to the trypanosome protozoa that causes African sleeping sickness, a killer disease that results when these organisms invade the human brain and central nervous system to cause meningoencephalitis.

Frank Richards was an expert in the generation of antibody diversity, the process by which our immune system "learns" how to make an antibody that is specific for almost any new invading pathogen in order to provide us with immunity. Frank noticed that there were interesting similarities between the human immune cells producing antibodies and the African trypanosomes. He and others found that trypanosomes produced many different parasite protein antigens (substances foreign to our bodies that evoke our immune responses) on their surface, known as variant surface glycoproteins (VSGs). The VSGs allowed the trypanosome to evade our host immune system and ultimately to cause sleeping sickness. This process was exciting for me because it was one of the first instances in which scientists figured out at a molecular level exactly how parasites survive and reproduce in humans despite our highly evolved system for immune defense. The study of African trypanosomes and their VSGs was at the forefront of the brand new field of molecular parasitology, resulting in the first applications of the emerging science of molecular biology to the study of medically important parasites, and I felt that during the 1970s I was probably one of the few undergraduate students studying in this area. More or less, molecular parasitology was to become my scientific specialty for the next four decades.

I spent a good portion of my undergraduate career in Frank's laboratory, working day and night in between classes. As a Yale "MB&B" major (molecular biophysics and biochemistry) I was encouraged to be in the lab and to contribute to scientific publications. My inclusion as a coauthor on some of Frank's research papers on the biochemistry and molecular immunology of trypanosome VSGs was a highlight of my undergraduate career. And seeing my name among the authors of a scientific paper proved to me that I had made a crucial start toward my chosen scientific career. Frank was an extraordinary mentor, not only because he taught me how to be a serious scientist in the lab, but also because he was a role model for how to become a professor and to work well with colleagues. He also taught me a lot about the sociology of science, and he had a great vision for how to bring people of diverse backgrounds together in order to advance new scientific fields. Even after I left Frank's lab, we stayed in touch, and because of him I returned to the Yale faculty after completing my medical and scientific training. Frank passed away in 2011 at the age of 82—he was a lifelong friend and mentor. He made Yale University a very special place.

While at Yale I learned that an exciting new program had been recently created at Rockefeller University, one that allowed simultaneous PhD and MD studies with Cornell Medical College (now Weill Cornell Medical College) located next door on the East Side of Manhattan. Rockefeller University had been known previously as the Rockefeller Institute of Medical Research—it's an institution that has produced more Nobel laureates and Lasker Award winners on a per faculty basis than any other university in America. I graduated from Yale in 1980 to enter the Rockefeller-Cornell MD-PhD program.

I have written previously about this period in my life in an article titled "The Medical Biochemistry of Poverty and Neglect," referring to Rockefeller's Laboratory of Medical Biochemistry, headed by Professor Anthony Cerami [1]. Briefly, like Frank Richards at Yale, beginning in the late 1970s into the 1980s, Tony, together with four or five other Rockefeller professors, including the Nobel laureates Christian de Duve and Ralph Steinman, and George Cross, Miklos Muller, and William Trager, among others, began applying modern molecular methods to the study of medically important parasites. Tony

Cerami was also a visionary and someone who displayed tremendous courage in the way he approached scientific problems. "Courage" is not a word ordinarily used to describe scientists, but I think it applies to Tony because he was fearless in tackling new disease problems regardless of the technologies required to study them. He never shied away from studying a disease because he was not an expert in a particular technique or even field of study. His approach was to focus on a particular disease and try to develop novel and innovative interventions. Starting in the late 1970s, Tony began devoting part of his Laboratory of Medical Biochemistry to the study of tropical diseases and parasites. For this purpose he received special financial support from a new "Great Neglected Diseases of Mankind" (GND) program under the leadership of Drs. Kenneth Warren and Scott Halstead based at the Rockefeller Foundation [2]. Ken Warren was also a great champion for tropical medicine, and his GND program soon exerted enormous influence on the field.

This was a critical time in American science. The first genes had been cloned in the early 1970s, giving rise to a new revolution in molecular biology. I arrived at Rockefeller University in time to take part in some of the first applications of molecular biology to the study of parasites and other tropical disease pathogens. But in some cases the most important tropical pathogens were barely being studied. For example, while in the university library I read about human hookworm disease, including an article written almost 20 years previously by a retired Rockefeller professor and legendary field parasitologist named Norman Stoll, who labeled it "the great disease of mankind" [1, 3]. On further investigation, I could find virtually no modern biology being applied to the problem except by a handful of individuals, including Professor Herbert Gilles at the Liverpool School of Tropical Medicine and Professor Gerhard Schad at the University of Pennsylvania in Philadelphia. I began taking the train regularly to Philadelphia and established a lifelong friendship and collaboration with "Gerry," who passed away in 2009 at the age of 81. Together with Tony Cerami and Gerry Schad, and working daily with an assistant professor in the lab, Nguyen Le Trang, we launched efforts to develop the first human hookworm vaccine, a quest that 30 years later has resulted in the first series of clinical trials for that vaccine, and now several other vaccines for parasitic diseases [1, 4].

During the course of my MD and PhD studies I met Ann, and we were soon living together in graduate student housing at Rockefeller University, paying the wonderful rent of what I remember to be $44 per month. The MD-PhD program gave me a modest stipend to live on, which was supported by a unique Medical Scientist Training Program sponsored by the National Institutes of Health. Ironically, not yet having children, we had more discretionary income in those days than we did when I became a faculty member in the years to come! Although I worked hard, it was still a nice life. At the time I met Ann, she was working for *People* magazine in advertising. Ann had graduated from Smith College and moved to Manhattan to do something big and interesting. I think it was a more stimulating place during the 1980s than it now is. While today I sometimes think of Manhattan as an island of rich people, back then it still had some grit and some edge to it. We mostly loved doing simple things: walking in Central Park, the used book shops on Fourth Avenue and St. Mark's Bookshop in the East Village followed by pierogi and borscht at Kiev or Veselka, coffee at Café Reggio in the Village, sushi at East in Kip's Bay, Bagel Works on Sixty-Sixth Street and First Avenue near Rockefeller, the ubiquitous Greek coffee shops—their rice pudding or "cheeseburger deluxe"(the "deluxe" referred to a piece of lettuce and tomato)—or strolling up and down First Avenue with a pizza slice.

I graduated Rockefeller in 1986 and then Cornell Medical in 1987, completed a residency in pediatrics at Massachusetts General Hospital's Children's Service and Harvard Medical School, and landed back at Yale for my pediatric infectious diseases and molecular parasitology postdoctoral fellowship. During the 1990s, still at Yale but now a member of the junior faculty, I organized a unique laboratory devoted to the study of parasitic helminths with the possibility of leveraging those discoveries into developing innovative vaccines. I had the Yale machine shop make a sign with the title "Medical Helminthology Laboratory" and nailed it to the door of an empty laboratory in the Yale public health building on College Street. My new lab focused initially on human hookworm infection, extending some of the studies I had begun as a doctoral student. We also looked at additional opportunities to work on other parasitic and tropical diseases. In parallel, I was seeing patients as a pediatrician at the Yale–New Haven Children's Hospital. My lab remained linked to Frank Richards's laboratory located just upstairs—Frank had started this wonderful Center for Molecular Parasitology supported by the MacArthur Foundation—while my clinical activities were tied to the division of pediatric infectious diseases led by I. George Miller, one of America's leading virologists and clinician investigators. My life was busy and incredibly stimulating.

Our family was growing. Matt was born in Boston during my clinical pediatrics residency and Emy shortly after we first moved to New Haven. We were pretty poor financially but rented a pleasant house in the Westville section, a sort of a

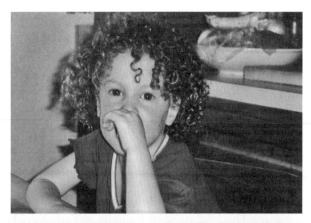

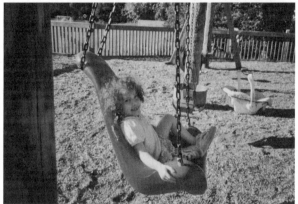

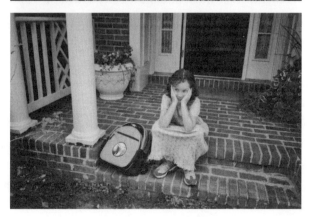

FIGURE 2. Rachel as a little girl in Cheshire, Connecticut

Yale faculty ghetto, before moving to Cheshire through the help of Ann's parents, who contributed to the down payment on a small house. We considered Cheshire a terrific place to raise a young family. I had the ideal job on the Yale faculty. Other than the fact that I was supporting a family of four on a very meager junior faculty salary, we felt we had made a comfortable and meaningful life for ourselves. We thought we had it all worked out.

Rachel was born in the fall of 1992. There was nothing particularly eventful about Ann's pregnancy with Rachel or the delivery at the Hospital of Saint Raphael at Yale–New Haven. Rachel was seven pounds at birth and grew up with striking red curly hair (fig. 2). The red hair was understandable, because my grandmother Rose Goldberg had red hair, and Ann also has red highlights. Ann was the first to notice something a bit unusual about Rachel compared with Matt and Emy. She often mentioned that Rachel was not as "huggy" as the other two. Most of her speech and physical developmental milestones were delayed, but not so alarmingly that we felt some type of intervention was needed.

Probably Rachel's most notable feature as a baby, besides not wanting to be hugged, was her loud and piercing cry, which in the beginning our pediatrician had ascribed to "colic." Ann remembers that Rachel would be consoled not so much by being hugged, but instead by lining up her toys in solitude on a table, the stairs, or a bookshelf and then dumping them on the floor. Rachel loved the repetitive motion of the swing, but otherwise when outside the house she would often try to run away. Rachel's elopements, colic, and crying made the house a much more stressful place than it had previously been. We remember that unlike the other children, Rachel was enormously difficult and not often very "fun."

When Rachel was 19 months of age, her pediatrician, Dr. Simone Simon, made referrals, first to a special "Birth-to-Three" program in Cheshire and then to the Yale child psychiatrists and their team at the Yale Child Study Center. One of the first American academic institutes devoted to child psychology and psychiatry, the Yale Child Study Center had been run by some of America's most important child psychiatrists, including Drs. Donald Cohen, Fred Volkmar, and Linda Mayes. Each of these psychiatrists would at one time or another wind up seeing Rachel, along with Dr. Wendy S. Levine, then a child psychiatry fellow, who would become Rachel's child psychiatrist for many years.

Rachel was diagnosed as PDD-NOS based on specific criteria according to a standard psychiatry reference known as the *Diagnostic and Statistical Manual of Mental Disorders*, fourth edition (*DSM-IV*). They include severe impairments in social interactions and communication skills, both verbal and non-verbal, and stereotyped behaviors and interests. Subsequently, in a revised *DSM-V*, the classification "PDD-NOS" was replaced with the more universal term "autism spectrum disorder" (ASD). But these diagnostic labels did not really tell the full story about Rachel. The Yale Child Study Center provided us with a detailed assessment of her abilities and deficits, with recommendations for a treatment plan. Ultimately, she performed poorly on tests of intelligence and behavior so that she was not even placed in a category of high-functioning autism previously known as Asperger's syndrome.

The title of this chapter, "Family Interrupted," reflects the life-changing ways in which our family adapted in order to keep Rachel living with us. Her elopement risk and negative behaviors made it difficult for us to obtain child care. Family trips became less and less frequent. And there were financial hardships. In order to manage Rachel and our family, Ann was unable to return to the workforce. It became a struggle to live in the northeast because of the high cost of living. Some recent estimates indicate that the costs of a child with ASD can be in the millions of dollars over a lifetime. In our view, that seems about right. And then there are the intangibles. Finances aside, it is and has been enormously stressful having Rachel in the house for the past 25 years. The full toll on us and her siblings remains to be fully determined.

Autism and Vaccines

As we were working out Rachel's diagnosis at the Yale Child Study Center, Ann and I began to hear a "buzz" about possible links between vaccines and autism. In 1998, Andrew Wakefield and his colleagues created a media storm and generated widespread interest following publication of their paper in the *Lancet* in which they reported a gastrointestinal syndrome associated with colitis and intestinal lymph node hyperplasia that was linked to "developmental regression in a group of previously normal children" who had received the measles, mumps, and rubella (MMR) vaccine [5]. Ultimately, that paper was corrected in 2004 and then retracted in 2010, more than a decade after it was first published. But the Wakefield paper helped to initiate a widespread belief that the MMR vaccine was causing an abrupt rise in autism or even an autism epidemic. The Wakefield hypothesis was subsequently followed by an alternative explanation put forward by others who claimed that autism or ASD resembled a form of mercury poisoning resulting from a thimerosal preservative contained in some childhood vaccines [6]. Still other theories purported that vaccines are being administered too closely together in time and somehow overwhelm the infant immune system, which might perhaps lead to ASD.

None of these hypotheses made a lot of sense in terms of explaining Rachel's autism or, indeed, any form of autism. Early on, meaning from the time Rachel was first diagnosed, it was clear to me that autism is a complex neurologic and developmental process or group of processes that must stem from alterations in the brain architecture and neurochemicals beginning way before birth. I felt that the complexities resulting in ASD could only be explained by genetic or epigenetic (how the genes are subsequently modified through biochemical and related processes or mechanisms) events before or immediately after the time of conception—in other words, way before infants ever receive their first vaccinations. If there is an environmental component to autism, it would have to be some type of prenatal environmental exposure.

Two decades after the initial publication of the Wakefield paper, a large scientific literature now refutes any links with vaccines. Numerous studies have more or less supported the genetic and epigenetic bases of autism and have outlined the role of these factors in creating changes in the brain of the fetus. The focus on prenatal development may also include the possibility that certain environmental exposures during early pregnancy might have some added role in the causation of ASD.

Despite the overwhelming scientific evidence that vaccines don't cause autism, an American and international anti-vaccine movement remains stronger than ever and is causing thousands of parents to stop vaccinating their children. The high rates of vaccine exemptions is now reaching a point where epidemic childhood infections once thought to be vanishing are now reappearing.

This book is about my passion for science and the science of vaccines (vaccinology) juxtaposed with the pseudoscience (and equal passion) of a robust, well-organized, and often aggressive anti-vaccine movement in the United States. It's about my effort to prevent an American-led anti-vaccine movement from derailing global gains in the fight against horrific, lethal, highly contagious, and highly preventable diseases. It's about Rachel, from a parent's point of view. I am a pediatrician, a scientist, and Rachel's father. And I can tell you, unequivocally, that vaccines do not cause autism.

· 2 ·

Saving Lives with Vaccines

After completing the MD-PhD program in New York, I was determined to pursue a life devoted to developing vaccines for neglected diseases such as hookworm. Because historically there was an intimate connection between vaccines and the field of pediatrics, it made the most sense to choose that area as a clinical specialty to complement my science. In June 1987, I became a pediatric house officer on the "Children's Service" (as it was called then) of the Massachusetts General Hospital in Boston. "MassGeneral" is one of the oldest and most distinguished hospitals in America, and its Children's Service began in 1821. Today the MassGeneral Hospital for Children is the oldest provider of pediatric care in Boston.

I spent two years as a MassGeneral pediatric house officer before heading back to Yale in order to specialize in pediatric infectious diseases. I remember my time in Boston for its steep learning curve, and I found it was not easy transitioning from the laboratory to the pediatric wards. During the 1980s, the MD-PhD program at Rockefeller and Cornell cut out the last year of medical school in order to allow completion of the whole program within seven years. Practically speaking, this meant a highly compressed timeline between finishing my doctoral dissertation at Rockefeller, completing my clinical rotations at Cornell, and then becoming a resident at the Mass-General pediatric emergency room in Boston.

One of the reasons I chose MassGeneral for pediatric training was its reputation for allowing its interns and residents quite a bit of autonomy. Back in the 1980s, the place sometimes projected a "sink or swim" kind of ethos. In fact, my attending physicians at MassGeneral at that time were referred to as "The Visit," meaning the house officers ran the show and the senior attending docs—well, I guess they visited! Having so much responsibility as a first- and second-year house officer forced me to learn how to make difficult—sometimes life or death—decisions and to live by them. Although a little frightening at first, ultimately the MassGeneral Hospital provided me with a lifetime of leadership skills. I'm pretty sure things are quite different there now, just as they are at all residency training programs across the United States. There's a much longer runway for stepwise increases in clinical responsibility and a much higher degree of supervision and oversight. Today, attending physicians known as "hospitalists" are in place around the clock, and the emergency departments and intensive care units have 24-hour senior attending physician coverage in most cases. This change followed some well-publicized legal cases at US hospitals in which it was alleged that some terrible patient outcomes occurred as a result of inadequate resident house staff supervision. So while the new system probably does help to ensure patient safety, I wonder if it also means that residents who graduate from house staff training programs are less self-reliant, self-confident, or ready to assume leadership responsibilities than in the past.

Hib

The late 1980s was a particularly interesting time to be a pediatric house officer or pediatrician in the United States because it represented a transition period when we saw the disappearance of a form of bacterial meningitis caused by invasive *Haemophilus influenzae* type b (Hib) infection in young children. Hib meningitis is a terrible illness that can result in long-term and devastating neurological deficits, including hearing loss, in children who survive the infection. Invasive Hib also causes other severe forms of illness, including epiglottitis (swelling of the flap of cartilage and tissue that protects the windpipe during swallowing), which could literally asphyxiate a young child within a period of hours. Meningitis and epiglottitis, as well as other invasive complications due to Hib, remain an important cause of death worldwide, causing almost 60,000 children to lose their lives annually. The species name, *Haemophilus influenzae*, of the bacterium is a bit of a misnomer. Around the time of the great influenza pandemic of 1918, some researchers thought Hib was the cause of flu until it was later realized that it represented a common complication of the illness. But even without previous influenza, Hib is itself a highly invasive and scary infectious disease.

As a pediatric house officer, I saw and learned firsthand how Hib meningitis could devastate children and their families. It mostly occurred in infants, toddlers, and other young children, and usually resulted to their admission to the MassGeneral pediatric intensive care unit (PICU). When I was working in the pediatric emergency department, infants and toddlers would sometimes arrive in a coma or having seizures. Once we got the seizures under control, I would then perform a lumbar puncture (sometimes known as a spinal tap) in order to examine the cerebrospinal fluid under a microscope and then bring it to the microbiology laboratory in order to culture the bacteria. To this day I still remember the sickening feeling I had when the cerebrospinal fluid would come out of the lumbar puncture needle white and cloudy, indicating that it was highly likely the child had a case of bacterial meningitis. In that case, I would immediately look at the cerebrospinal fluid under a microscope we had in a backroom of the MassGeneral emergency department. After staining the sample, I could see the characteristic shape and color of Hib bacteria in and around a microscopic field of white blood cells.

Once bacterial meningitis was suspected, the pediatric house officer on call in the emergency department would proceed immediately to administer intravenous antibiotics. If the child was sick enough, a team would come down to the emergency room to provide measures for maintaining life support, including intubation, before placing the child on a respirator or breathing for the child through a handbag, and sending the child to the PICU. From there it was mostly a waiting game to determine if the child awoke and could have the breathing tube removed, followed by a very prolonged and agonizing recovery process that could last months. Permanent neurological deficits were common, and sometimes the child did not make it and died.

As you can imagine, the emotional toll on the parents and families was immense. Hib meningitis also took an emotional toll on the MassGeneral pediatric house staff. It was a horrible disease, made even more horrible for me because my first son, Matthew, had been born when I was a MassGeneral house office and was at about the age when he was susceptible to Hib meningitis. My Hib patients were mostly about my new son's age. That I might bring Hib home from the hospital and infect him became my single greatest fear. At that time and into my pediatric infectious diseases fellowship, it was recommended that if you had close exposure to a Hib patient, you should take a drug called rifampin as a form of prophylaxis to prevent self-infection or transmitting Hib in the community. The medicine had a side effect of turning one's urine red-orange in color. It seemed as if I lived with orange urine in those days.

But then a miracle occurred. Figure 3 is a graph from the Centers for Disease Control and Prevention (CDC) showing the annual incidence of invasive Hib disease in children under the age of five and how the number of occurrences changed with time. Before 1985, invasive Hib disease was one of the leading causes of meningitis in the United States and caused approximately 1,000 deaths annually [1, 2]. The incidence showed a sudden small drop between 1985 and 1987. And then, after I became a house officer in 1987, the decline accelerated. Five years later, when I was an assistant professor of pediatric infectious diseases at Yale University School of Medicine, Hib was mostly gone, and I would teach about invasive Hib meningitis and epiglottitis for its historical interest. By the mid-1990s on the wards at Yale–New Children's hospital, I would speak to the pediatric house staff about Hib in the same way that my MassGeneral attending physicians used to talk to us about diphtheria or measles.

So what happened? Why did invasive Hib disease disappear? The answer is that a first-generation Hib vaccine became available in 1985, which was subsequently refined and improved and licensed in 1987. During the 1970s, Drs. Porter Anderson and David Smith, working at Boston Children's Hospital, isolated a capsule of Hib that contained polyribosphosphate and demonstrated that it could be used as a vaccine that would elicit protective antibodies [3]. This work led

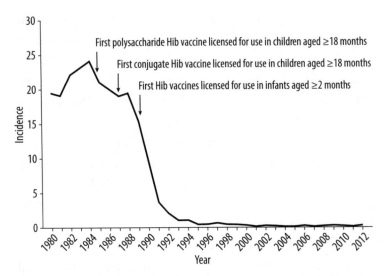

FIGURE 3. Estimated annual incidence (per 100,000 population) of invasive *Haemophilus influenzae* type b (Hib) disease in children aged under five years in the United States, 1980–2012.

Source: Briere EC, Rubin L, Moro PL, Cohn A, Clark T, Messonnier N; Division of Bacterial Diseases, National Center for Immunization and Respiratory Diseases, CDC (2014). Prevention and control of *Haemophilus influenzae* type b disease: Recommendations of the advisory committee on immunization practices (ACIP). MMWR Recomm Rep. Feb 28; 63(RR-01): fig. 1.

to the licensure of this first Hib vaccine in 1985 [3, 4]. Subsequently, Drs. John Robbins and Rachel Schneerson at the National Institutes of Health improved the polysaccharide vaccine by showing it could be conjugated to a protein backbone [4]. That advance made the Hib vaccine much more effective in toddlers and young children under the age of two—the population that needed it most. The US Food and Drug Administration first licensed this vaccine for children older than 18 months in 1987, and then for infants in 1990. Today there are only about 40 cases of invasive Hib disease occurring each year in the United States.

As a young pediatric house officer in Boston, and later as an attending pediatrician at Yale, the Hib vaccine was for me the most visceral and tangible example of the power of a vaccine—a tool that could eliminate a devastating disease over the course of just a few years.

American Vaccines: A Success Story

The United States has been fortunate to see similar drops in infection rates for a variety of diseases, indeed for most of the diseases for which we now vaccinate children. For example, a quick search of the CDC website or the biomedical literature reveals similar and dramatic down curves or drops for measles, mumps, and rubella after those vaccines were introduced during the 1960s [5], and even earlier declines following the widespread use of vaccines for diphtheria, pertussis (whooping cough), and tetanus [5–8]. More recently, the rotavirus vaccine was introduced in the United States in 2006, and now more than 40,000 hospitalizations are prevented annually [9]. The introduction of the pneumococcal conjugate vaccine (PCV) has resulted in similar successes.

The decision by CDC to introduce new vaccines such as the rotavirus vaccine or PCV to prevent pneumococcal pneumonia is made in consultation with an interesting organization known as the Advisory Committee on Immunization Practices (ACIP), which celebrated its 50th birthday in 2014 [10]. Although ACIP is focused on US policies and practices and has been involved with almost every major American vaccine decision during the past five decades, over time ACIP has also had important international influences. Many nations now also adopt policies established by ACIP, which makes its decisions on the basis of both vaccine effectiveness at preventing disease, as well as cost-effectiveness [10]. The policy role for ACIP really expanded beginning in the 1990s when the United States established an entitlement initiative known as the Vaccines for Children (VFC) program, which provides an important safety net to ensure vaccine coverage in this country [10]. The program provides ACIP-recommended vaccines free to all children who are uninsured, and these vaccines are now also part of the preventive services of the Affordable Care Act (ACA) [10]. ACIP wields prodigious power, since its recommendation has enormous implications for these two health programs. In order to ensure the independence of ACIP, no federal employees can serve on the committee, and the director of the CDC can no longer chair the committee. More recently, the financial relationships between ACIP members and the vaccine manufacturers have been called into question, and there is an ongoing effort to monitor and address any actual or perceived conflicts of interest [10]. For the anti-vaccine community, this is a major point of contention. Many of their arguments rely on conspiracy theories surrounding the CDC and ACIP, a topic that I will return to later.

With the exception of pertussis and breakthrough measles epidemics, most of the terrible and killer infectious diseases have gone the way of invasive Hib infection and have mostly disappeared in the United States. Nationally, the CDC has determined that 14 diseases have disappeared or could soon disappear. In one of its recent public service announcements it names them the "14 diseases you almost forgot about (thanks to vaccines)" [11]. Today, the United States has an outstanding system in place for ensuring access to vaccines for the vast majority of the human population. Specifically, children living in financially stressed or vulnerable families have access to vaccines through the VFC program [12].

The 14 childhood diseases currently targeted by vaccines recommended by the CDC include diphtheria, tetanus, and pertussis (through a combined vaccine that's abbreviated DTaP); Hib, pneumococcal disease, and rotavirus infection; measles, mumps and rubella (through the MMR vaccine); hepatitis A and B, varicella, flu (influenza), and polio [11]. For preteens and teens, additional vaccines are recommended to prevent cervical cancer and meningococcal disease, among others. It has been noted, however, that adolescent populations present a special challenge, because at least four vaccines are newly recommended—Tdap (an adolescent/adult version of the combined vaccine for tetanus, diphtheria, and pertussis) meningococcal conjugate vaccine, cervical cancer, and regular influenza vaccines [12].

Many of these vaccines were first developed in the academic or industrial laboratories (or both) of American scientists, including those against Hib, rotavirus, measles, mumps, rubella, and polio, during the 1950s through the 1980s. Therefore, the dramatic reductions in deaths from childhood infectious diseases in America were pioneered through government, academic, and industry partnerships. Such partnerships first began in the year before America entered World War II. In a recent article published in *Scientific American*, I credit leading scientist-administrators from MIT, Harvard, and the Carnegie Institute, including Vannevar Bush, who successfully persuaded President Franklin Roosevelt to co-invest in science along with increases in funding to scale up the military and security. This military-academic-industrial complex created a revolution in American science not only for vaccines, but also in physics, computers, chemistry, and engineering [13].

Increasing Successes Globally:
Smallpox Eradication and the Expanded
Program on Immunization (EPI)

Beyond US borders and throughout the 1960s and 1970s, we also began to observe a sea change and uptick in vaccination rates and vaccine coverage globally—even in some of the world's poorest nations. From my perspective, a key stimulus for launching vaccinations on a global scale was the smallpox eradication campaign that began in 1966. In that year, Dr. Donald A. (DA) Henderson moved from the CDC to Geneva in order to head this initiative at the World Health Organization (WHO). Although smallpox had been eradicated from the United States by 1950, during the 1960s it was still a leading global killer, causing possibly as many as two million deaths annually, but also producing permanent disfigurement in many other cases [14, 15]. At that time, smallpox and measles were leading the race for killing the world's children. DA was an extraordinary field marshal who led an amazing group of public health experts and scientists—including Drs. William Foege, Larry Brilliant, and Ciro de Quadros. Together they established a unique system of "ring vaccination" in which the smallpox vaccine was specifically targeted to family members or household contacts of known smallpox cases. Another major advance that enabled an eradication campaign based on vaccination was the ability to create a freeze-drying process for the smallpox virus that allowed its transportation in hot and tropical countries. It has been noted that this process was pioneered by Soviet scientists, so smallpox eradication actually represents a sterling example of what I term "vaccine diplomacy" between Cold War foes [16].

Owing to the efforts of these dedicated medical professionals and scientists working over the course of 11 years under incredibly harsh and unforgiving conditions in some of the most difficult places on earth in terms of terrain, climate, or conflict, the last naturally transmitted smallpox case occurred in Somalia in East Africa in 1977. Smallpox became the first disease to ever be completely eradicated—an accomplishment that ranks at the top of achievements in the history of medicine [14, 15]. During his lifetime DA Henderson received the National Medal of Science and the Presidential Medal of Freedom [15]. After eradicating smallpox, he also became the dean of the School of Public Health at Johns Hopkins and was later recalled out of retirement in order to help the administration of President George W. Bush build a response to global bioterrorism in the wake of 9/11 and the anthrax attacks in Washington, DC, and elsewhere [15]. But what I remember with special fondness is the time when DA spent a morning in my office when I was a young microbiology department chair at George Washington University, wanting to learn everything he could about our efforts to develop vaccines for neglected tropical diseases. That was one of the most memorable days of my life.

As the smallpox campaign was winding down, it was clear that an important global vaccine infrastructure had been built in order to deliver vaccines in remote and isolated areas. Rather than let it lie fallow, WHO was able to leverage this global health system in order to deliver additional vaccines. In 1974, WHO created an innovative Expanded Program on Immunizations (EPI), which delivered the BCG (bacille Calmette-Guérin) vaccine for tuberculosis, in addition to vaccines for diphtheria, pertussis, tetanus, polio, and measles in the first year of life [17]. Later, booster doses of polio and other vaccines, and of course the smallpox vaccine, were provided [17]. The initial progress was slow, but EPI provided proof of concept that it was possible to create a health system for delivering vaccines. EPI ultimately laid the foundation for a revolution in childhood vaccination coverage through a new global alliance.

Gavi, the Vaccine Alliance

EPI was an inspirational program and one that achieved unprecedented coverage of childhood vaccines. But there was room for improvement. Beginning in the early 1990s and following the World Summit for Children in New York, a new Children's Vaccine Initiative (CVI) was proposed, which would be supported by an alliance of partners that included the Rockefeller Foundation and several United Nations (UN) agencies such as WHO, UNICEF, and the World Bank [18]. The basic goal of CVI was to significantly expand existing EPI global immunization coverage for the six vaccines targeted toward the world's poorest countries while simultaneously building on the growing science of vaccinology in order to develop new vaccines for existing and emerging global health threats, including rotavirus, pneumococcus, meningococcus, and cholera, as well as HIV/AIDS, malaria, and tuberculosis [18, 19]. At the time CVI was being proposed during the 1990s by Dr. Philip K. Russell and others, I was already an assistant professor at Yale. The concept of CVI was an important inspiration for me to persevere in my efforts to develop the first human hookworm vaccine. Although, for reasons detailed by the public health historian Bill Muraskin, CVI did not achieve its aspirational goals [19], it still provided a foundational basis for convening global leaders to create a new initiative, which at the dawn of the twenty-first century became one of the most important and successful of all of the global health initiatives.

In 2000, two major initiatives were launched. The first was known as the eight United Nations Millennium Development Goals (MDGs), which were established by the UN Secretary General in order to sustain poverty reduction for the poorest people on the planet living on less than $1 per day. One of the most important goals—MDG 4, to reduce child mortality—focused global attention on how child deaths reinforced poverty and, consequently, the need to scale up vaccinations for the world's children as a highly cost-effective measure for saving lives.

The second proposal in 2000 was to establish a new and effective Global Alliance for Vaccines and Immunization (GAVI), later rebranded as Gavi, the Vaccine Alliance. Gavi became the enabling mechanism to implement goals and targets linked to MDG 4. Like CVI, Gavi also brought together international stakeholders, including the major UN agencies, and was intended to address a global concern that 30 million children were not fully immunized annually with the EPI vaccines [20]. Gavi would help push to get EPI to the next level in terms of both expanding vaccine coverage and introducing new vaccines for Hib, rotavirus, and pneumococcal disease [21].

From my perspective, a key game changer in making Gavi successful (whereas CVI fell short) was the Bill & Melinda Gates Foundation. In 2000, the Gates Foundation provided an amazing $750 million in seed money, which made it possible for Gavi to effectively seek co-investments and regular replenishments from prospective donor countries. It now had the resources to begin the job. Another important piece for ensuring Gavi's success was its innovative and flexible structure that facilitated the creation of private-public partnerships that brought together multinational pharmaceutical companies, developing-country vaccine manufacturers, governments, and

TABLE 1. Selected causes of global deaths for both sexes combined in 2015, with percentage change between 2005 and 2015

Disease	Childhood deaths (under age five) in 2015	Percentage change, 2005–15
Pneumococcal pneumonia	393,000	–38.8
Rotaviral enteritis	146,500	–43.6
Measles	62,600	–75.1
Haemophilus influenzae type b	58,700	–60.7
Pertussis (whooping cough)	54,500	–41.0
Tetanus	25,500	–57.2
Diphtheria*	2,100	–61.3
All causes	5.82 million	–27.2

Source: From tables 5–7 in GBD 2015 Mortality and Causes of Death Collaborators (2016) Global, regional, and national life expectancy, all-cause mortality, and cause-specific mortality for the 249 causes of death, 1980–2015: A systematic analysis for the Global Burden of Disease Study 2015. Lancet 388: 1459–544.

*Includes both children and adults.

the UN agencies highlighted above. In so doing, Gavi was able to donate vaccines free of charge or significantly reduce the cost of vaccine prices and create an infrastructure that made it straightforward for low- and middle-income countries to receive or purchase the essential vaccines. Gavi estimates that between 2000 and 2016 (the 2000–2015 lifespan of MDG 4, plus one additional year), more than 640 million children received access to essential vaccines and 9 million lives were saved [20]. By 2020, an additional 5–6 million deaths may be prevented and 300 million additional children vaccinated [20]. There is no question that Gavi represents one of the greatest public health success stories of this new century.

But we do not need to rely exclusively on Gavi's own reporting to measure the impact of expanding childhood vaccination coverage. That's because, in addition to helping to launch Gavi, the Gates Foundation also created an organization known as the Institute for Health Metrics and Evaluation based at the University of Washington, Seattle, for evaluating changing patterns of disease prevalence and incidence. This is happening through an activity known as the Global Burden of Disease Study (GBD). GBD is a massive undertaking that involves hundreds of investigators globally. Over the past few years, I have helped GBD in its assessments of neglected tropical diseases. Under the leadership of Dr. Christopher Murray, the studies conducted by the GBD are being published in a series of capstone papers in biomedical journals, with major summary articles in the *Lancet* [22]. For example, table 1 presents a list of the major infectious killers of children under the age of five for the year 2015, but it also shows the reductions in mortality between the years 2005 (when Gavi was well under way) and 2015, the year that MDG 4 was completed [22].

Overall, the numbers are incredibly impressive and really highlight the power of vaccines. They show that while hundreds of thousands of infants and young children still die of vaccine preventable diseases, led by pneumococcal pneumonia, enteritis caused by rotavirus, measles, invasive Hib disease, pertussis, tetanus, and diphtheria, those deaths declined dramatically during the decade spanning 2005 and 2015 [22]. Most notably, there was roughly a 40 percent decrease in deaths as a result of vaccination with the two new vaccines introduced by Gavi (PCV and rotavirus vaccine, respectively) and about a 60–70 percent reduction in deaths in most of the childhood diseases thanks to expanding coverage of the older

EPI vaccines. I consider such numbers indicative of a slam-dunk success story, such that Gavi could be considered the single most important initiative financed so far by the Gates Foundation. These numbers are also critical for ensuring that Gavi funds are replenished by the US government or indeed the other group of seven (G7) countries.

In 2017, Gavi, currently under the leadership of Dr. Seth Berkeley, reported additional and impressive figures and accomplishments [20, 21]. Since 2000, Gavi's accomplishments in terms of saving lives have occurred through expanded use of a pentavalent vaccine to prevent diphtheria, pertussis, tetanus, invasive Hib disease, and hepatitis B; vaccines for pneumococcal pneumonia, rotavirus enteritis, yellow fever, and Japanese encephalitis; the measles, mumps and rubella (MMR) vaccine with the addition of a second measles vaccine dose; and meningitis caused by meningococcus group A [20, 21]. Almost one-half of those deaths were averted just between 2011 and 2015 [21]. Gavi has also strengthened health and immunization systems and services in dozens of countries and created systems for introducing new vaccines.

Beyond saving lives, Gavi has generated impressive economic returns on investment while dramatically reducing vaccine cost [21]. Gavi has also helped to build capacity for manufacturing vaccines in the developing countries of Africa, Asia, and Latin America, so that countries in these regions do not have to rely on vaccines being shipped from North America or Europe [21].

Despite these enormous successes, we still have a long way to go for Gavi to complete its mission. Gavi and WHO estimate that 1.5 million children still die globally from vaccine-preventable infections, while less than 10 percent of children in Gavi-supported nations receive all of the vaccines that currently are recommended by WHO [21]. Some of the worst-performing countries in terms of under-immunizations include those affected by conflict or political instability—Afghanistan, Chad, Democratic Republic of Congo, and Pakistan—although a few of the very large low- and middle-income countries such as Indonesia, Nigeria, and Pakistan are also underachieving in terms of providing vaccine access [21].

To further address such disparities, Gavi has an ambitious plan to continue expanding vaccine coverage. The approaches include expanding country co-financing and capacity building to transition dozens of additional countries away from their dependence on Gavi. The key message is that vaccines work; we're making stunning progress in terms of reducing global child deaths; and if we can remain on this trajectory, we could reach a point where children no longer die from a vaccine-preventable disease.

A Mostly Noncompliant Little Girl

There was nothing particularly eventful about Ann's pregnancy with Rachel. Ann was 32 years old at the time; it was her third pregnancy, and things more or less went according to plan. A look back at Ann's medical records reveals that her pregnancy was normal. Her water broke (rupture of membranes) about 12 hours prior to delivery. Rachel Kate was born as a full-term baby at the Hospital of Saint Raphael at Yale–New Haven on October 14, 1992. She weighed 3.3 kg, or just over seven pounds, and had excellent APGAR birth scores (a general assessment of newborn well-being) of 9 at one minute after delivery and again 9 at five minutes. In every respect this was an ordinary birth process and happy occasion. Emy (three years old at the time) was excited to have a little sister, as was Matt (then, almost five years old).

The first few months of Rachel's life seemed relatively normal in terms of her development, or at least compared with that of the two older kids. At two weeks of age, Rachel did have an elevated temperature that was just above 100°F and was noted to be irritable; after a full medical work-up, she was admitted overnight to Yale. At that time both of her siblings also had a flu-like illness with respiratory symptoms, so most likely it was some upper or lower respiratory virus infection. By the next morning she was well enough to return home.

Perhaps more significantly, Ann did note that Rachel as an infant did not feel the same as Matt and Emy. For example, after Daniel, our younger son, was born, four years after Rachel, Ann told me that in infancy Rachel did not "mold" to her contours the way Dan did. I think it's helpful to hear in Ann's own words about Rachel's first few months:

> Rachel's body had a different feel when I held her. She felt stiff and not relaxed from the time that she was a very young infant. I put that feeling on hold, as I was extremely busy caring for now three small children. Our household was chaotic but happy, as I remember, and we tried hard to give each child personal time with us, if only for brief periods of time. Chores and child care were my focus then and for many years to come.
>
> Rachel's piercing cries could be heard up and down Buttonwood Circle in Cheshire, as I tried to calm her down. She was about two months old and it was colic, we were quite sure. Ear infections, persistent colds, and digestive problems all could have contributed to her distress. Doctor's visits confirmed mild illnesses and we carried on.

Ann kept all of Rachel's immunization records. Rachel received all of her scheduled vaccinations as recommended by the CDC and ACIP. Over the first few years of life, beginning when she was two months of age, she received five doses of the combined diphtheria, tetanus, acellular pertussis (DTaP) vaccine, and then boosters in 2006 for tetanus and diphtheria (Td), and later in 2011 for all three diseases (Tdap)—the adolescent/adult formulation. She also received the two scheduled measles-mumps-rubella and varicella vaccine doses, and four doses each of the polio vaccine and Hib vaccine. Rachel received three doses of the hepatitis B vaccine and also her hepatitis A vaccine, meningococcal vaccine, and HPV cervical cancer vaccine. To this day she receives annual influenza vaccines.

Early Intervention, Child Psychiatrists, and a Pediatric Neurologist

During her first year, Rachel's growth was basically normal, but she was behind the other kids in terms of when she sat unsupported (at nine months instead of six months). Other than that, we hadn't noticed a lot in terms of developmental delays. However, by 18 months of age we became very concerned that Rachel was not walking or talking. In Ann's words:

What a relief it was when Rachel was not crying! She was older now, about five months, and she was intensely interested in a handful of small cardboard books that babies are first presented with. *Goodnight Moon, The Runaway Bunny,* and an alphabet book were particularly fascinating to Rachel. She is going to love books and be a great reader because she has an amazing attention span, I remember thinking. She was content to sit in her car seat, in the dining room or another quiet place and read. Not once did I imagine that there were any other issues at play.

Visiting with our wonderful pediatrician, Dr. Simone Simon, was generally a time to ask any question during our checkups, at which time we received a prescription for amoxicillin or some timely advice about car seats or perhaps a cream for eczema. At the 18-month checkup, quiet concern was observed. Dr. Simon simply stated that Rachel was not reaching the typical milestones for a child that age. Had Peter and I not noticed this before?

She did not pose that question, but we did. How could it be that Peter, a pediatrician himself, and I, an experienced mother, hadn't noticed? I think we had seen differences, but we attributed them to what we knew, or thought we knew, about child development. Children do not all learn and grow in the same ways, or at the same speed.

How did I miss it? Matthew was four and a half and Emy was three when Rachel was born. I tried to be an amazing mother to all three, and yet there was almost never enough time to focus on any one child. I must have known that I wasn't bonding to Rachel, that strong connection wasn't there, but I didn't want to consider what that might mean. I knew nothing about autism and it was all very frightening for me. Basically, I tried to fix whatever problem was in front of me at the time, and I protected myself by not thinking too deeply.

A whirlwind of phone calls and appointments with several specialists (including an audiologist), teachers, and social workers followed Dr. Simon's first referrals, and our life was changed forever from that time on.

Rachel's visit to Dr. Simon prompted a referral to the Birth-to-Three intervention team at the Darcey School in Cheshire. Darcey serves both as a kindergarten in the Cheshire public school system, as well as an early intervention and special needs center for the town. By the time Rachel was 20 months of age, she was starting to talk, but the Darcey team noted that "there were significant delays in all areas." These time frames for diagnosing Rachel's developmental delays are fairly classical for ASD. We've since learned that they represent a period when important changes to the structure of the brain have been noted in kids with the disorder. Specifically, a group at the University of North Carolina (UNC)–Chapel Hill found that significant overgrowth in brain volume is under way between 12 and 24 months of age [1]. Brain volume overgrowth is emerging as an important manifestation linked to the symptoms of ASD. The UNC–Chapel Hill team has also determined that even though brain volume overgrowth coincides with initial signs of ASD, the process is actually initiated at least a year earlier [2]. Later we'll see why this information is important in understanding why vaccines don't cause autism.

The Darcey School early intervention program was excellent. It was a beautiful and welcoming environment with caring and professional teachers who were kind and generous with their time. Ann believed they were truly gifted and felt lucky that all of the services required could be provided right there. Rachel attended school five hours a day, five days a week. Even a summer program was provided. She received twice weekly sessions for both speech and language services, as well as occupational therapy. (I recognize that kids don't have occupations in the usual sense, but they are expected to progress in certain skills, including play.) In Rachel's case, in order to benefit from speech and language therapy, she needed to be placed in a calm and quiet room with minimal distractions. Typically, one skill would be worked on at a time, with an emphasis on repetition until that skill was mastered. There was also lots of positive reinforcement through use of language. On the "occupational" side, however, Rachel's fingers were weak, and she could barely pick up a crayon except to throw it across the room. You could not simply present her with a crayon or writing instrument and expect her to produce anything of interest. The staff at Darcey devoted much time to trying to get her to hold her crayon and draw a line from one place on a page to another. To provide reinforcement and make it interesting, the occupational therapists would help Rachel to focus by providing her with different textures, such as sand, water, and intriguing types of shapes and screens.

By the time Rachel was 29 months old, however, she was functioning at the 18-month level in most areas, and she was especially rigid and scripted in her social conduct. She would often repeat the same questions or phrases over and over. For example, I remember her often saying, "The camel has two humps." In the spring of 1995, Rachel was first referred to the Yale Child Study Center, when she was seen by Dr. Wendy S. Levine and diagnosed with PDD-NOS. Dr. Levine noted that Rachel was "limited in her imaginative play, has difficulties in social relatedness, and is often quite anxious." She also observed that Rachel was "easily overwhelmed by stimuli, and can become scattered motorically, running about randomly."

In addition to starting play therapy, several different treatment regimens of psychiatric medicines were attempted, but each one seemed to be worse than the other. Prozac was too activating, Zoloft was too sedating, Luvox increased aggression, while Risperdal did not result in any improvement. Finally, Rachel was taken off psychiatric medicines entirely and is currently not on medication.

At five years of age she had formal IQ testing, which confirmed our worries that not only was Rachel diagnosed with PDD-NOS, but she had significant intellectual disabilities. A few results stood out. First, there was a big disparity between her verbal and performance IQs; and second, despite her verbal strengths, she still had major problems in that area. Although her verbal IQ score was 84, which approaches a normal range, she would not speak expressively but rather tended to repeat phrases she had heard. In Rachel's second year of life, after months of grunting, her first word was "Cheerios," a cereal she still eats almost every day as an adult, and quickly thereafter she began speaking in complete sentences. But the content mostly included phrases that she had heard on TV or in passing conversations. She would repeat entire dialogues from the *Power Rangers* or *Teenage Mutant Ninja Turtles* but would not say "I love you mommy" or "Look at the pretty flowers." Far worse was Rachel's performance IQ, which measures nonverbal skills and required her to engage in specific tasks. On this Rachel scored quite low at 60, and her full-scale (total cognitive capacity) score was 69. Her later IQ testing was not even this high, in some cases going down to the 40s in the performance area.

As part of an extended Jewish family that deeply values intellectual abilities and accomplishments, these findings were especially difficult for Ann and for me. Ann initially was not accepting of the diagnosis of PDD-NOS or the low level of intellectual ability, and she initially responded with disbelief. She would pore through the *DSM-IV* to find alternative diagnoses, and there was lots of intellectualization. In the end, what was so devastating for us was not really the autism component, but instead it was the low level of intellectual functioning. It took years, but over time we came to an understanding that Rachel would have a very different life from what we had hoped for her. We faced a real possibility that she would not find a life partner, attend college, or have a meaningful career. There was a lot of sadness and sense of loss.

On top of the sadness, taking care of Rachel had become grueling. More mobile, she began running away from home, ignoring our shouts to return. She had no sense or understanding that she was placing herself in dangerous situations.

She would go up to strangers constantly to start conversations, and in odd ways. In stores, for instance, Rachel would either routinely walk up to older men and say "Hi, grandpa," or she would query customers about the contents of their shopping carts. In clothing stores or supermarkets, Rachel would go off and hide, sometimes mobilizing the entire staff to try to find her. Marshall's became our special horror. We learned that it can be really challenging to locate a child within dozens of racks of clothing.

As a child Rachel liked to dump things—on the floor, in the toilet, or out windows (including windows of moving cars), whether it was food or toys, and later, schoolbooks and homework assignments. It was noted by staff at Darcey and the Yale Child Study Center that she would do so with "impulsivity" and "excitement." At this age, Rachel seemed to obtain some type of gratification from extreme reactions or our being upset. The greater our reaction or emotional response, the more she would smile or laugh. Fishing items out of the toilet bowl was a regular occurrence. We learned not to open the back car window on the side where Rachel had her car seat. Eventually we had to learn to mute our responses as a way of reducing the likelihood that Rachel would engage in destructive or impulsive behaviors. We can't say for sure that this approach was effective.

She was a mostly noncompliant little girl. Rachel would seldom listen to us, and if she did so, it was only after multiple reminders or warnings. "[S]he is heedless of her parents' limits," wrote one of her therapists. "Her parents can usually only get her attention by physically containing her or being sure she is looking directly at them." One technique that Ann learned would sometimes work was to sit on the floor, placing Rachel between her legs while they looked at books or toys. Another technique was driving in the car with Rachel strapped in a car seat, which became times when Ann would engage her in conversations. The repetitive motions of playground swings were also effective in that regard.

Rachel was also extremely rigid or compulsive, engaging in an identical routine and eating the same seven or eight foods day in and day out—Cheerios, Rice Krispies, toast, yogurt, shredded cheese, pasta with Prego brand tomato sauce, pizza, and Kellogg's Nutri-Grain bars. She would watch taped videos of cartoons on the VCR, but she preferred to play the same one over and over again until she had memorized most of it. A favorite cartoon was about a brother and sister who traveled in space and time. Every morning and afternoon we would hear the mom on TV exclaim, "My baby in another dimension? Do they feed you up in space?" while the kids would respond, "Not really." Twenty years later, our whole family can still recount the dialogue in detail.

There was little imaginative play and very few social interactions with peers. To address this aspect we spent two years doing play therapy at the Yale Child Study Center, in addition to working with Rachel's Darcey teachers. There were modest gains and improvements, but they were incremental compared with the rapid or exponential gains of her siblings when they were the same age. In addition, Rachel was often emotionally labile and would easily cry, and when she did, it was often loud and piercing. At this age, there were very few times when Rachel would spontaneously express love or affection toward us. In its place and with us Rachel was mostly interested in objects, animals, or engaging in negative behaviors. She did have a sense of humor, especially slapstick humor, and Rachel enjoyed it when I would speak for her stuffed animals and engage them in ridiculous conversations. But these were short-lived moments.

For the most part, taking care of Rachel alternated between being dreary or frightening. As Ann and I would often say to each other, she's "hard as hell." Looking after Rachel was wearing us down. Our exhaustion was compounded by the fact that she seldom gave much back emotionally, compared with the other children. Eventually we consulted both Drs. Linda Mayes and Fred Volkmar, two of the giants of ASD child psychiatry research at Yale. Dr. Volkmar was a lead author of the autism section of the *DSM-IV* and served for several years as the director of the Yale Child Study Center. Dr. Mayes has a long and distinguished history while also serving as director. When Rachel was six years old, she had an evaluaton on Winchester 1, the inpatient child psychiatry unit linked to the Yale Child Study Center. As part of the evaluation she underwent an EEG (electroencephalogram) that revealed an interesting finding of some right-sided temporal lobe spike discharges, for which she received tegretol for a time, possibly with some improvement. But doing blood draws to assess tegretol levels became a monumental task because of her noncompliant behavior, and eventually it got to the point where it appeared tegretol had stopped producing any tangible benefits.

Ultimately, Rachel went on to have two psychiatric admissions to Winchester 1. They confirmed an interesting disparity or split between her verbal skills, which were below average but still close to the normal range, and nonverbal skills, which were profoundly low. Aside from PDD-NOS, one of Rachel's other early diagnoses included nonverbal learning disability syndrome, a diagnosis that is also not used much today, but at that time Rachel was quite verbal, so her psychiatrists felt this added label was useful. Today both of these identifications have been subsumed under the category of ASD.

In order to help Rachel, the team of psychiatrists at the Yale Child Study Center recommended programs of intense behavioral interventions in school and at home. Carrying this over to the home was easier said than done. We began to rely more and more on other adults and teenagers in the neighborhood to help with the two older kids, so Ann could focus on Rachel. We wanted Matt and Emy to have a full and interesting life, which eventually included extracurricular activities, including sports. Matt became a pretty good ice hockey player, so we had to become a hockey mom and dad of sorts. Emy was doing figure skating, soccer, and was very involved in art—she also became an excellent writer. Over time, Ann developed a support network. It included Michelle, a teenager living across the street who had lots of creativity and innovative ideas for the older children. Snow days and school cancellations were pretty common in Cheshire, and those could be exhausting and demoralizing times with Rachel. Michelle frequently came to our rescue on those occasions to help with Matt and Emy. Dr. Laurie Sheiner, a pediatrician who worked at Connecticut Children's Hospital, became a good family friend and helped out enormously. Two college graduates, Chrissie and Kate, were hired to help out with Rachel, and Ann's mother, Marcia, made heroic trips from New Jersey on a weekly basis. But overall, our safety net with Rachel was rather fragile and fragmented.

In the meantime, my work in parasitic and neglected tropical diseases began to require significant travel overseas, and on top of it all, by this time I had received funding for a large NIH-supported Tropical Medicine Research Center (TMRC) program project in China, which required me to be in Shanghai at that city's Institute of Parasitic Diseases. The genesis of the project was interesting. China had recently conducted the world's largest survey of human parasitic diseases, and it was found that during the early 1990s, literally hundreds of millions of Chinese suffered from parasitic infections. I was privileged to not only develop vaccines for hookworm and other parasitic diseases in my laboratory, but during my early career at Yale I had the opportunity to help lead a team of international scientists to better understand why China had so much disease and how to control it. Together with my international colleagues Professors George Davis, David Blair, and Donald McManus, each a global expert on parasitic worm infections, we were one of the first teams to have the opportunity to conduct a "deep dive" into the parasitic and tropical diseases across the poorest parts of China. Working at anti-epidemic stations in remote areas, we got to see a part of China that few westerners ever saw. The stakes were high because by then China had made plans to build a dam across the Yangtze River in order to help meet the vast hydroelectric demands of its rapidly expanding and industrialized population. However, this new Three Gorges Dam would create water reservoirs that could potentially further promote a rise in the number of cases of schistosomiasis and other parasitic diseases. We were on the front lines to investigate such possibilities.

That was the exciting part. The not so exciting part was that the work required me to make regular trips to China and leave Ann behind with the children. During each trip I had to live with a fair amount of guilt that I was abandoning Ann for a week or two at a time. But it was not to last. On one of my China visits, Rachel required a second psychiatric hospitalization at Winchester 1. I wound up taking more than 24 hours of different flights to Shanghai for one full day of meetings and then returned home on the next flight out. Almost fifty hours of travel for one working day of meetings. I don't recommend it.

The fallout was that I had to start making choices, which included restricting my travel in order to preserve the family. It was a great professional disappointment, but I had to gradually phase out my activities in China and focus on regions closer to home. Over time I had to pivot away from Asia and turn my attention to parasitic and neglected diseases and health disparities in the Americas. In a sense, I could "commute" to Brazil or Panama by leaving on a Monday and returning on a Thursday and thus remain at home on weekends. Even if I went into the lab or office on a Saturday or Sunday, at least I was around and home for dinner.

· 4 ·

Derailment

As the global public health community geared up to vaccinate the world's children through Gavi, the Vaccine Alliance (under the auspices of the UN's Millennial Development Goals in the early 2000s), a counterforce was also beginning to take shape. During this period a new or "neo" anti-vaccine or anti-vaxx (anti-vax) movement was beginning in the United Kingdom, Europe, and ultimately the United States.

The First American Anti-vaccine Movement

Our current situation, which began in 1998, is not the first time that anti-vaccine attitudes have threatened the health and safety of Americans. Anti-vaccine movements have been around in one form or another since the founding of the American colonies. The Reverend Cotton Mather was a Massachusetts Puritan minister who sometimes got it right, but at other times he came out on the wrong side of history. Mather was a proponent of the Salem witch trials but was also arguably America's first great vaccine champion.

Smallpox, also known as variola, caused deadly and widespread epidemics in New England during the late seventeenth

ANTI-VAX, ANTI-VAXX, OR ANTI-VACCINE?

It's common to use any of the three terms "anti-vax," "anti-vaxx," or "anti-vaccine." The anti-vaccine movement often uses "vaxxed" to refer to bad things that happen to kids who receive vaccines, while the pro-vaccine community often uses the term "anti-vax" or "anti-vaxx" in a disparaging way. When I'm interviewed on TV or radio or for newspapers, my wife generally admonishes me against using the term "anti-vaxx" because she feels it's pejorative and unnecessarily provocative. With journalists, I sometimes lapse into using "anti-vax" or "anti-vaxx" when I'm frustrated or angry with those opposed to vaccination, but ultimately I think she's right. So for this book, "anti-vaccine" wins, at least most of the time.

century and early 1700s. The disease was probably introduced through trade across the Atlantic, and aside from mandatory quarantine of ships coming into Boston Harbor, the colonies had very few weapons to fight it. Rev. Mather had other ideas. Possibly from one of his African slaves, he learned about the practice of scraping a pustule from a smallpox patient and then inoculating this infectious material (that contained living smallpox virus) into another individual so as to induce a mild form of the disease. This immunization practice, known as "variolation," could in many cases prevent smallpox. In unimmunized individuals smallpox was associated with approximately 30 percent mortality. Almost a century later, Sir Edward Jenner replaced variolation—scraping a human smallpox lesion—with vaccination (from the Latin, "cow"), which involved scraping a cowpox lesion (although some allege that the virus contained in smallpox vaccine more closely resem-

LEISHMANIZATION

There is a truly ancient form of immunization that predates variolation. Cutaneous leishmaniasis is a disfiguring infectious disease of the Middle East, North Africa, and Central Asia. It is caused by single-celled Leishmania parasites and transmitted by sand flies. Today it is still known as "Aleppo evil" and "Baghdad boil," among other names. The ancients figured out that scraping an active lesion and inoculating it on the buttocks or limbs of an individual, frequently a child, could prevent a natural infection that might result in facial disfigurement and social stigma. Today, the Texas Children's Hospital Center for Vaccine Development is developing a next-generation leishmaniasis vaccine using genetically engineered recombinant proteins from the parasite and sand fly.

bles horsepox). Vaccination proved to be a much safer and superior technique, which ultimately enabled a next-generation smallpox vaccine used for global eradication efforts. But even in the early 1700s, variolation proved to be an important advance in protecting Boston from the threat of smallpox.

The Boston smallpox epidemic of 1721 was a devastating one, in which hundreds of people perished. Indeed, the smallpox epidemics of the early 1700s were among the most deadly in American history, especially for Native American populations, who were highly vulnerable. But when it came to smallpox prevention, Mather was a visionary. He was an early proponent of variolation and successfully persuaded his physician colleague Dr. Zabdiel Boylston to begin variolating hundreds of individuals. (When Ann and I lived in Boston during my pediatric residency in Boston we lived not far from Boylston Street.)

This period also ignited the first major American anti-vaccine movement. In response to variolation pamphlets written by Mather and his proponents, some local newspapers objected, while other area physicians wrote countervaccine pamphlets condemning the practice. Some suggested that variolation violated natural laws put forth in the Bible and other religious writings [1]. Things reached their nadir when the objectors to vaccination tossed some sort of homemade bomb into Mather's home. Appended to the device was a note that read, "Cotton Mather you dog, dam you! I'll inoculate you with this; with a pox to you" [1]. (Such a story reminds me that perhaps I should complain less about the snarky or even mean-spirited e-mails, memes, and tweets that I receive from my anti-vaccine critics!) Ultimately, the Mather-Boylston variolation campaign may have worked. It has been estimated that the death rate from variolation was around 2 percent, whereas mortality in the Boston smallpox epidemic exceeded 14 percent [1]. In recognition of his achievements, the Reverend Mather was made a Fellow of the Royal Society of London.

Since that time, American anti-vaccine sentiments have never completely disappeared. During the early twentieth century, for example, the renowned physician Sir William Osler spoke out against the "anti-vaccinationists." Osler, who held posts at McGill University and Oxford, is also an important and historic figure in modern American medical practice. Along with the pathologist William Henry Welch, the surgeon William Stewart Halstead, and the gynecologist Howard Kelly, he helped to found the Johns Hopkins School of Medicine, considered by many the first modern medical school in America.

However, by the middle of the twentieth century America turned decidedly in the pro-vaccine direction. During the 1950s, polio caused devastating childhood summer epidemics in major US urban centers, and parents lived in constant fear of the disease during those times. Clinical trials on a polio vaccine developed by Dr. Jonas Salk began in 1954 and included more than one million American schoolchildren, comprising more than 400,000 who were administered the vaccine and negative control groups that received either a placebo vaccine or no injection at all. Results of this massive nationwide study were revealed on April 12, 1955, and demonstrated that the Salk vaccine was more than 90 percent effective. Salk was hailed as a national hero and placed on the cover of *Time* magazine. The widespread acclaim that Salk received for his polio vaccine development efforts reveals how much the American population appreciated his discovery. Indeed, the decades following World War II probably represented a golden age when the public celebrated vaccine developments and were quick to line up in order to ensure their children received new vaccines that had become available [2].

Dark Clouds: Vaccines and Autism

When exactly did the modern anti-vaccine movement based on alleged and specious links to autism begin? Fortunately, through the US National Institutes of Health (NIH) and its National Library of Medicine, we can trace the origins with some precision. Throughout the 1980s, when I was in medical and graduate schools, and even into the 1990s, whenever I needed to look up a topic in the biomedical literature, I would go to the *Index Medicus*, a voluminous series of encyclopedic books that listed papers appearing in most of the major journals by topic. Then in 1996, in a ceremony led by Vice President Al Gore, PubMed came online. PubMed is a free and open access online computer search engine that covers all of the information from

Index Medicus but also allows links or even access to articles across the universe of the rapidly expanding biomedical literature. Today, from the comfort of my home or work, or while I'm traveling, I can search PubMed for almost any topic published in the biomedical literature over the past half-century, or sometimes even further back. If the journal is "open access," such as one of the Public Library of Science (PLOS) or BioMed Central journals, you can even download the full article free of charge. Since 2007, I have served as founding editor in chief of *PLOS Neglected Tropical Diseases*, the first open access journal for these illnesses.

Today, a PubMed search using the phrase "vaccines and autism" reveals some interesting findings. The first paper that comes up is a small article in a German pediatric journal from 1976 that reports on a 15-month-old boy who showed signs of autism (then known as Kanner Syndrome) a few weeks after receiving his smallpox vaccination [3]. (Remember that age, because we're going to come back to it.) The article indicates that a causal relationship is "unlikely," but it set into motion a far more influential article some 20 years later, which in my opinion launched the modern anti-vaccine movement as we know it today.

For more than the next 20 years, the biomedical literature was silent about vaccines and autism. Then, in 1998, Andrew Wakefield and his colleagues, based at the Royal Free Hospital and School of Medicine in London, published a paper in the *Lancet* on 12 children (11 of whom were boys) who ranged in age from 3 to 10 years and were referred to a specialized unit for pediatric gastroenterology [4]. The major physical complaints of the children were abdominal pain and diarrhea, together with deficits in language and developmental milestones that resembled autism or ASD [4]. The parents or physicians of

eight of the children noted that their regressive behaviors began within days or weeks after receiving a dose of the measles-
mumps-rubella (MMR) vaccine.

Each of the children enrolled in the study received extensive
workups that included magnetic resonance imaging, lumbar
punctures, and endoscopy of their colons and ileums, in addition to intestinal biopsies. Wakefield and his colleagues noted
that the 12 children exhibited abnormalities in their intestines,
with 11 showing evidence of chronic inflammation in their colons. There was also a proliferation of gut lymphoid tissue noted
in seven children. Nine of the children had autism [4]. The authors clearly implied that all three major pieces—MMR vaccination, colonic inflammation, and neurodevelopmental delays
or regression—were somehow linked to produce a single disease or syndrome culminating in autism. Their major conclusion was that they had discovered "a unique disease process."
The authors' final statement sums up their major findings as
follows: "We have identified a chronic enterocolitis in children
that may be related to neuropsychiatric dysfunction. In most
cases, onset of symptoms was after measles, mumps, and rubella immunization" [4]. Today, PubMed lists more than 700
papers using the words "vaccine and autism" as subject head-
ings, with all but one of them appearing after the publication
of the Wakefield et al. paper in 1998. That manuscript launched
a new field of inquiry.

In 2010, more than a decade after the original publication,
the *Lancet* fully retracted the Wakefield paper. In its published
retraction statement, the editors explained that the investigations approved by the local ethics committee were "proven to
be false" and that the children participants for the study were
not "consecutively referred," as the authors had claimed [4].
But the Wakefield paper and its retraction became a cause

célèbre, in part because of the sensational nature of the claims, but also owing to the diligence of Brian Deer, an investigative reporter for the *Sunday Times* (London) who specializes in medical issues. In the years leading up to the retraction, he filed a number of stories about the article and its authors. Then, in 2011, the lead editors of the *BMJ* (*British Medical Journal*) commissioned Deer to produce a series of articles about Wakefield [5–10]. Writing about Deer in a series preface published in the *BMJ*, the editors note that "it has taken the diligent scepticism of one man, standing outside medicine and science, to show that the paper was in fact an elaborate fraud" [5]. Summing up their allegations, the *BMJ* editors assert:

> [S]even years after first looking into the MMR scare, journalist Brian Deer now shows the extent of Wakefield's fraud and how it was perpetrated. Drawing on interviews, documents, and data made public at the GMC [British General Medical Council] hearings, Deer shows how Wakefield altered numerous facts about the patients' medical histories in order to support his claim to have identified a new syndrome; how his institution, the Royal Free Hospital and Medical School in London, supported him as he sought to exploit the ensuing MMR scare for financial gain; and how key players failed to investigate thoroughly in the public interest when Deer first raised his concerns. [5]

Off to the Races in England

Despite the eventual retraction of the *Lancet* paper and the debunking of Wakefield's alleged vaccine-autism links, a public health scare in the United Kingdom ensued and continues still [11]. Following publication of the Wakefield paper,

MMR vaccine rates dropped from over 90 percent to 80 percent between 1996 and 2003, while vaccine coverage in one area of London dropped to just above 60 percent [11]. Low vaccine coverage with MMR vaccine continued for years and remained about 10 percentage points lower than other childhood vaccines by the year 2006 [11]. Meanwhile, occurrences of measles began to increase, from 56 confirmed cases in 1998 to more than 400 in beginning of 2006, which included a measles death—something that had not happened in more than 14 years [11]. By 2008, measles transmission was noted to be sustained within the population of the United Kingdom and was described as "endemic." A 17-year-old with an immune deficiency disorder died that year of the disease [11]. In 2016, an additional 20 measles cases were noted in London, Cambridge, Essex, and Hertfordshire [12]. The elimination of measles in the United Kingdom had been reversed.

The European Continent

While measles was erupting in the United Kingdom, fears about the links between MMR vaccine and autism spread across the rest of Europe. By 2017, there were large numbers of unvaccinated individuals in about a dozen countries across Europe [13]. As of the summer of 2017, Romania and Italy were in the midst of a major outbreak comprised of thousands of cases and a significant number of deaths [13]. By the end of 2017 WHO estimated that Europe experienced more than twenty thousand measles cases and dozens of deaths. Elsewhere, in places such as Mongolia and some African countries, the year 2017 was shaping up to be a bad one for measles [14].

The rise of measles epidemics in Europe is due to the drop in vaccine "coverage," meaning the percentage of children in a community who receive their measles vaccine at one year of age or who receive a second dose before school entry. Once measles vaccine coverage falls, we can expect measles outbreaks to appear. This is because measles is one of the most highly contagious viruses known. A single individual infected with measles can on average infect more than a dozen unvaccinated children, especially infants under the age of one, who are not yet old enough to get vaccinated [15]. Practically speaking, this high rate of contagion means that once vaccination rates go below 90 to 95 percent, we see measles [15]. Such is the situation we currently face in Europe. We can reliably expect to see significant European measles outbreaks in the coming years.

A Second Line of Attack

Just as the mainstream medical community was beginning to mount a measured and scientifically based response to the hypothesis of Wakefield et al., a second theory arose alleging a different vaccine-autism association. In a paper published in 2001 in the journal *Medical Hypotheses*, a group proposed that autism represented a form of mercury poisoning related to a mercury-containing preservative found in some vaccines, known as thimerosal [16]. Thimerosal, or ethylmercury (also known as Merthiolate), is an organomercury antiseptic used in a variety of medical products and even in tattoo inks. Prior to 2001 it was also used in a large number of pediatric vaccines, especially in vials with multiple doses. The rationale for adding thimerosal to a multi-dose vial is that each time a needle is introduced to withdraw an amount of vaccine, it can also potentially introduce bacterial contamination. Bacterial contamination of vaccines was an important problem that needed to be addressed. During the early twentieth century, bacterial contamination in batches of typhoid and diphtheria vaccines in South Carolina and in Australia, respectively, led to bacterial abscesses at the site of injection and even some deaths [17]. Adding thimerosal preservative reduces this likelihood, and it was selected as a preservative after studies showed it inhibited bacterial growth at extremely low concentrations and did not alter the ability of the vaccines to induce a protective immune response, sometimes referred to as vaccine "potency" [17]. By the 1940s, thimerosal was used in a variety of biological products such as vaccines and serums [17]. It was an important advance that was considered a breakthrough in terms of immunizing large populations, especially in resource-poor settings.

However, the authors of the paper in *Medical Hypotheses* noted how mercury exposures and poisoning can cause neurological and behavioral deficits, a few of which can bear resemblance to autism. For example, Minimata disease, named after a city in Japan, resulted from a chemical plant's industrial release of a methylmercury form of mercury (different from thimerosal) in wastewater that accumulated in a bay where fish and shellfish lived and were consumed as seafood. Large-scale methylmercury ingestions in pregnant mothers caused a congenital syndrome, causing neurologic disease in the form of gait and motor disturbances that in some cases resulted in coma and even death. Although autism is not typically associated with gait or motor abnormalities like Minimata disease, a new allegation arose that the ethylmercury component of thimerosal may also produce something bad, possibly a variant of Minimata disease in the form of autism.

To complicate matters, the groups alleging the thimerosal-autism link further suggested that vaccines were causing a unique type of ethylmercury poisoning, but only in a subset of individuals who are genetically predisposed to injury from this type of environmental toxin. Robert F. Kennedy Jr., a prominent environmental attorney and son of the deceased US Attorney General Bobby Kennedy, became passionate about this problem and edited a book on the role of thimerosal that recommended the "immediate removal of mercury" from vaccines [18]. Together with "Mercury Moms," a parent group that created an organization known as Safe Minds [17], Kennedy Jr. has campaigned aggressively about the harmful effects of mercury and their alleged autism links [18].

Although the US Food and Drug Administration (FDA) found no evidence that thimerosal in pediatric vaccines was causing harm, it nonetheless recommended that the compound should be removed and that pediatric vaccines should be made thimerosal-free [19]. In 1999, two years prior to the publication of the *Medical Hypotheses* article, the FDA made its recommendation because of both the feasibility and the desirability of reducing overall infant mercury exposure, rather than any proven links to autism. In the United States, removal was achieved largely by reformulating pediatric vaccines in single-dose vials. Today, all routine immunizations for children under the age of six are provided using vaccines that do not contain thimerosal preservative [19, 20]. Despite vaccinating children with thimerosal-free vaccines for many years now, the rates of autism have remained unchanged. Some people allege that autism rates have *increased*. Such findings are borne out through additional studies conducted in both Scandinavia and California. If thimerosal was indeed responsible for ASD, we would expect rates to eventually diminish.

Thimerosal has been removed from all pediatric vaccines used in the United States, with one exception: influenza vaccines. Most of the FDA-approved single dose vaccines for children are now thimerosal-free, although one known as Fluvirin still contains "trace" amounts (less than 1 microgram of per 0.5 ml dose). In addition, multi-dose flu vaccines used for adults (including pregnant women) and children still contain 25 µg of thimerosal. Accordingly, some groups have advocated banning use of multi-dose flu vaccine vials for use in pregnancy, even though, as we will see later, at least one major study has not found any association between maternal flu immunization and autism among children.

"Green Our Vaccines"

In 2007, yet a third line of attack was opened on vaccines. A California-based pediatrician, Dr. Robert Sears, wrote a book that became a best seller. *The Vaccine Book: Making the Right Decision for Your Child*, by "Dr. Bob" (as he is sometimes known) proposes alternative immunization schedules based on an erroneous belief regarding the harmful effects of delivering too many vaccines at once. He outlines a plan to spread out vaccines gradually in order to avoid what is sometimes called "antigenic overload" or overwhelming an infant's young immune system [21, 22]. There are multiple problems with such recommendations. First, the vaccine schedule promoted by Dr. Sears goes against established recommendations from the CDC, the American Academy of Pediatrics, and ACIP. Without clinical trials in place to evaluate the alternative schedule, it's quite possible or even likely that the alternative approach will not be effective or as effective as the recommended regimen. Also, the idea that an infant's immune system could somehow be overwhelmed by an infant vaccine series has few, if any, scientific underpinnings and ignores the fact that an infant's gastrointestinal and respiratory tracts represent highly effective organ systems for introducing multiple new molecules in the environment as antigens. An infant's immune system is likely stimulated by dozens or even hundreds of new antigens daily, so the idea that we're somehow overloading it with a few vaccine antigens makes little sense to me. It has also been pointed out that the 14 major vaccines now given actually contain fewer antigenic components than the 7 vaccines given during the 1980s, not to mention the fact that autism is essentially a change in neurodevelopment and not a disease of the immune system [23]. Nevertheless, the alternative schedule proposed by Dr. Sears has found enough acceptance among parents and parent groups such that today it is not uncommon for parents to request delays in the vaccine schedule or to withhold it altogether. Such requests are contributing to gaps in vaccine coverage.

Shortly after the Sears book was published, the celebrity community began to weigh in. In 2008, Jenny McCarthy and Jim Carrey marched on Washington, DC, with a demand to "green" vaccines by removing thimerosal or other toxic substances in vaccines or to space them out. Dr. David Gorski, who is a surgical oncologist at Wayne State University but also an editor of *Science-Based Medicine*, elucidated the issue eloquently: "[I]t should be apparent that the 'Green Our Vaccines' slogan is nothing more than putting an eco-friendly face on antiscientific fear mongering in the cause of opposition to vaccines" [24].

Aluminum

Many of our childhood vaccines are formulated with aluminum salts, such as aluminum hydroxide or aluminum phosphate. Sometimes referred to as "alum," these aluminum salts help to concentrate the active ingredients of the vaccine in a "depot" once they are injected in the muscle. In so doing, they help to activate our immune system in order to respond to the vaccine [25]. The immune stimulating properties of alum have been known since the 1920s [25], such that it is one of the oldest and most tested components found in human vaccines. Today, alum is an essential component for several commonly used vaccines, including the diphtheria-tetanus-acellular pertussis vaccines, pneumococcal conjugate vaccine, and hepatitis B vaccine [26], as well as the human papillomavirus (HPV) cervical cancer vaccine. Some of the neglected disease vaccines that we are developing, such as those for human hookworm infection and schistosomiasis, are also formulated on alum and are now in clinical trials [27]. To date, there is no evidence that alum-adjuvanted vaccines cause autism or ASD in humans, although there are several studies purporting to link alum or alum-adjuvanted vaccines to social impairments and biomarkers related to autism in mice. However, two of those studies were subsequently retracted [28].

Caught Off Guard

The anti-vaccine movement launched by the 1998 *Lancet* paper in the United Kingdom spread not only to Europe but to the American side of the Atlantic Ocean. This community does not usually speak with one voice. The Wakefield camp alleges that MMR links to autism; while others, such as Robert Kennedy Jr., implicate thimerosal; and Dr. Robert Sears and Jenny McCarthy recommend spacing or withholding vaccines. Still others have raised new challenges such as aluminum contained in some childhood vaccines, or that there is just something unsavory about vaccines that requires us to "green" them. Increasingly, I have been confronted by journalists or those in the anti-vaccine community about my role as a vaccinologist and my efforts to refute the Wakefield-RFK-Sears-McCarthy assertions. I became frustrated, because each time I whacked down one allegation, a different one popped up.

As the anti-vaccine movement began to gain momentum beginning in the early 2000s, I for the first time found myself needing to actually defend the safety and integrity of vaccines. I had become a vaccine scientist because I saw it as one of the highest expressions of science in the pursuit of humanitarian goals, but now in response to queries from the media, and even some friends and colleagues, I had to justify why I was trying to develop vaccines for diseases of the poor. I felt something had gone terribly wrong. Could it be that the amazing vaccine train (which was saving so many lives) had somehow derailed?

It did not take me long to realize that the problem was not the science. The science told me not only that vaccines saved lives, and millions of lives at that, but also that vaccines were safe. In addition, although at that time we were still on a steep learning curve about the causes of autism, it did not seem plausible to me that a vaccine could cause this condition. After all, Rachel's behaviors were incredibly complicated, and Ann had noticed something different about Rachel since birth (prior to ever receiving her childhood vaccinations), even though she was not finally diagnosed until her second year of life. My mind could not formulate any molecular or other mechanism by which an immune response to a vaccine would produce the complex changes in the cellular architecture of the brains of children on the autism spectrum.

Instead, I began to feel that the anti-vaccine movement was off the mark. Many of those expressing anti-vaccine sentiments were shrill and often angry, and at times unwilling to listen to my reasons why vaccines did not or could not cause

autism. It was a movement whose members were mostly un-
concerned with scientific evidence, or if they were, they would
be selective and piece together fragments of facts to construct
a pseudoscientific narrative. At times I came to believe that
the anti-vaccine proponents were not always interested in getting to the truth, but were merely expounding on their beliefs,
almost like a religious cult. In my opinion, this was a tremendous waste of useful energy, which could be better directed
toward more productive endeavors such as finding ways to
help families like mine with both autism and mental disabilities. I came to believe that the anti-vaccine movement was a
destructive force.

· 5 ·

Like Rome during the Roman Empire

In 2000, our family relocated to the Washington, DC, area for my new job as an academic department chair at George Washington University (GWU). GWU gave me a remarkable opportunity to build a new microbiology and tropical medicine department in its medical school, with a large amount of space in a building located just a few blocks from the State Department, the Pan American Health Organization, and the White House. My research group had just received new funding from the Bill & Melinda Gates Foundation to develop our human hookworm vaccine and bring it to the clinic. We were also able to leverage the Gates funding in order to advance a second vaccine for schistosomiasis, another devastating parasitic disease. We now had a team of scientists developing the first-ever vaccines for these diseases, a quest I had begun as an MD-PhD student in New York. In so doing, we were pioneering the idea of developing a vaccine in a nonprofit and academic laboratory.

But another attraction of GWU was that it was in Washington, DC, during a very interesting time—"like Rome at the height of the Roman Empire"—I would tell my colleagues. Working and living in the nation's capital opened an entirely new public policy and advocacy dimension to my work. In addition to heading our work in the laboratory, I now had a foot firmly planted in public engagement and science policy, and I began to advocate for taking on a variety of parasitic and tropical diseases affecting the poor.

Wider Horizons

The year 2000 was an important one for global public health because that was when the United Nations' Millennium Development Goals (MDGs) were launched. The MDGs represented an international effort to address the plight of an estimated one billion people living in extreme poverty (on less than one dollar per day), a group that at the time was known by some as the "bottom billion" in reference to a book with that title written by Paul Collier, an Oxford University economist [1]. The MDGs became a framework for international development assistance in order to lift people out of poverty. They were adopted by the United Nations member states and provided a road map for the UN agencies, such as UNICEF and the World Health Organization.

In all there were eight MDGs, three of which linked poverty to health. MDG 6 was written "to combat AIDS, malaria, and other diseases," and this goal prompted the Bush White House to launch the President's Emergency Plan for AIDS Relief to help provide large populations in Africa, Asia, and elsewhere with antiretroviral drugs, as well as the President's Malaria Initiative, in addition to a Geneva-based Global Fund to Fight AIDS, Tuberculosis, and Malaria. The only problem with this goal was that it left out all the other diseases, including the parasitic diseases that I was studying previously at Yale and now GWU. In response, I teamed up with two esteemed colleagues (and friends) from the United Kingdom, Professors David Molyneux and Alan Fenwick, to shape a concept that we named "the neglected tropical diseases" (NTDs) that branded a group of 13 to 14 chronic and debilitating parasitic diseases, like hookworm infection and schistosomiasis. We also identifed a "rapid impact" package of drugs that could be used to target these diseases, which could be delivered for only 50 cents per person annually [2, 3]. Together, the three of us also enlisted the help of international economist Professor Jeffrey Sachs, Dr. Lorenzo Savioli at WHO, Dr. Eric Ottesen, and other colleagues, and then approached the White House and US Congress [4]. Because I was already working in the heart of Washington, DC, it often fell to me to lead US government advocacy efforts, which eventually resulted in funds for the package being appropriated in order to launch a new NTD Program at the United States Agency for International Development [5]. The end result is that almost one billion people have now been treated with partial or complete NTD packages, representing one of the world's largest public health programs.

Rachel's Adolescence

Still another reason for relocating to DC was to be close to Ann's sister Julie, who could help with all the kids and spend time with Rachel, now an adolescent. However, there were challenges with the move. The Washington suburb of Rockville, Maryland, unlike Cheshire, is really a small city and a very hectic and busy place. For our family the move was definitely a transition to a faster-paced life. Another challenge we faced, however, was that it was nearly impossible to find a child psychiatrist like Dr. Levine in the DC area, especially one that took our health insurance. There's no question that our nation has a dearth of child psychiatrists, and not nearly enough to deal with the huge numbers of kids now being diagnosed with ASD. We were able to have Rachel seen by Dr. Mark Batshaw, who serves as chief academic officer at the Children's National Medical Center in Washington. Mark is also a distinguished developmental pediatrician, and he noted the disparity between Rachel's verbal and performance IQs. He also identified important components of her behavior that resemble attention deficit hyperactivity disorder (ADHD), and oppositional defiant disorder (ODD). Mark further noted her odd sleep patterns, in which she was up much of the night but exhausted by the afternoon. Such traits are not uncommon with ADHD, and it is still an issue with Rachel to this day.

Rachel first attended the Carl Sandburg Learning Center in Montgomery County, close to where we lived in Rockville, and then the Montgomery Village Middle School and the Forbush School at Oakmont Upper School. Her ASD was considered "atypical" in that she had strong verbal skills. It's interesting to note that this trait is an important new trend being noted with increasing frequency among girls with autism, who are clearly on the ASD spectrum and yet often display better verbal and social skills than boys. Although not as well known in the early 2000s, there is now an expanding scientific literature about girls with autism, who are often noted to be better socialized than boys and yet retain much of the rigidity and other features on the autism spectrum. It's been also reported that girls with ASD have high rates of comorbidities, such as eating disorders, obsessive-compulsive behaviors, and even features resembling ADHD. Certainly, Dr. Batshaw had picked up on some of those trends.

At the age of 12, Rachel was evaluated at the Carl Sandburg Learning Center. Psychological testing administered by

Dr. Seth Goldberg at that time confirmed her previous discrepancies in scores, including a verbal IQ of 87, but a performance IQ of 49. We had seen disparate scores before, but we had never seen such a profoundly low performance IQ. Ann was especially devastated and questioned its validity. It's certainly true that to this day Rachel cannot tie her own shoes, or do simple puzzles, or even perform simple math such as addition or subtraction or counting of money or change. Yet Ann still does not understand how Rachel could have so few performance skills given her verbal talents, and how personable Rachel can be on some days.

Dr. Goldberg is an impressive psychologist who made the following evaluation:

> Rachel continues to present, as she approaches the end of her elementary school career, as an autistic spectrum youngster, who presents with one of the most fascinating and intriguing patterns of strengths and needs, even in a program geared to the needs of complex, multiply handicapped children. . . . Rachel is both outgoing and emotive. On the one hand her letting you know how she feels is very useful in being able to support her. On the other hand Rachel is capable of becoming flamboyantly melodramatic, and so narcissistically involved in her own perceptions of what is going on around her, that she is capable of lavish displays of inconsolable sadness, that can really only be disrupted after a while by withdrawing attention from her.

Indeed, Rachel often acted out whenever she was presented with a challenge that was too hard. Requiring her to remain on task or do schoolwork frequently produced disruptive behavior that would get her out of the class. Unless it was a topic that was on Rachel's priority list, such as the Power Rangers or certain types of animals, she would either become extremely loud and disruptive, or use foul language. Rachel could speak like a truck driver when the occasion demanded. She knew how to manipulate people to get her way and get out of tasks. Alternatively, she would feign clinical symptoms and walk herself to the nurse. We always dreaded a call from the school nurse, because it meant Ann had to drive back to the school, pick up Rachel, and bring her home. It signified another lost day.

"Rachel has real verbal/cognitive skills to use for learning, and an enormous fund of environmental information gleaned from the rich experiential life that she lives outside of school, as well as her books, television programs, and movies that she brings to bear in learning situations in the school setting," wrote Dr. Goldberg. In this sense, some of Rachel's teachers found her to be interesting and even endearing. One of Rachel's favorite TV shows then (I'm sorry to say) was *Yo Momma*, in which two opposing parties would try to insult each other's mother, with credit given to the most clever insult. Rachel memorized some of these insults to great fanfare among the students and teachers. Sometimes she would forget the second half of the joke and would ad lib some ridiculous things about someone's mother.

The assessment continues:

At the same time Rachel's needs continue to emanate from both cognitive and interpersonal inadequacies. Her pragmatic language for learning is less than fully adequate to deal with curricular issues. She has, as I have said, a very limited range of interest. Her actual social skills to engage in friendships and interactions with other children are likewise limited by her autistic status, and her difficulties self-monitoring, and applying braking mechanisms to her own emotional and behavioral responses, in order to keep functioning within acceptable bounds. Rachel can display high levels of cognitive rigidity and an inability to deal with redirection or negative feedback in instructional situations. She continues to have a great deal of difficulty coping with curriculum content that is abstract and non-experiential, that has to be grasped on a verbal/conceptual level. Also, as she moves into her adolescence, Rachel may be even more prone to oppositional and task avoidant behaviors when threatened by task difficulty or complexity and so shake her self-concept and self-confidence.

Indeed, Dr. Goldberg was prophetic. Beginning in middle school and throughout high school, Rachel would hide in the bathroom from her special needs teachers, and to this day when confronted with a new or intimidating situation, she will take off for the bathroom or other venue. Such avoidant behaviors have also prevented her from gaining meaningful employment. At one point we were advised to create a structured summer environment by having Rachel spend several weeks at a camp in the Poconos dedicated to special needs. Rachel not only hated it but also refused to eat the food. Essentially, she went on a hunger strike, and we had to pick her up early and take her home. Dr. Goldberg also noted, "At the same time, Rachel has a lot going for her, given her disable [sic] status. Rachel has lots of experience trying to cope with and fit into the social set of non-disable children, outside of school and the experiences that are provided for her by her parents. Although she will strike other adolescents as very different and will need a lot of support, so as not to behave in ways toward potential friends that are incursive or annoying. . . . Difficulties early in Rachel's tenure should be anticipated."

Some of Rachel's teachers liked her and enjoyed working with her, but at least an equal number found her challenging because of her noncompliance and the fact that she had a "loud voice" and would frequently "argue with the staff." Such behaviors became especially evident later during her high school years. She would sometimes spend half the day in the ladies' bathroom using her phone. When confronted by teachers, Rachel would also spit and swear, which was a new development. While such behaviors can also be associated with tics and Tourette-like syndromes in some kids with autism, we had the sense that this was different and of a voluntary nature. The school ultimately worked out a strict behavior chart for Rachel, which included when she could go to the ladies' room.

Rachel also objected to any kind of form-fitting clothing. She refused to wear a school uniform or would do so only after extensive arguments. In some sense, she had replaced the older negative behaviors such as putting things in the toilet, running away, and dropping objects out of moving car windows with a new set of avoidant or oppositional behaviors. Because of my heavy travel schedule, Ann bore the brunt of dealing with so many of these complications.

Although her handwriting was extremely poor and barely legible, Rachel was able to read at a reasonable level. She enjoyed using Google and reading about Justin Bieber or certain boy bands such as One Direction, or she would research different zoos around the world. She knew every major zoo in every major city. Eventually she enjoyed hearing about new restaurants, especially fast food restaurants, and would read menus online. The computer became an outlet for her latest obsessions, which have included the Power Rangers, Alvin and the Chipmunks, the *Fast and Furious* movies, One Direction, and some Japanese anime. Ann and I scratched our heads to try and find a common denominator to Rachel's interests.

Unfortunately, if asked or required to read a book on a topic not of her interest, she would pronounce it "stupid" and refuse all pleas and attempts to get her interested. For example, her teachers wanted her to read *Tom Sawyer* or other children's classics, or something called "Brain POP" that covered various aspects of science, math, or social sciences. Forget it, it was not on Rachel's radar screen. Ann recalls the general tenor of these times:

> I am trying to be positive here, but Rachel's school days were hard for her as a student, and almost as hard for me as her parent. Having a daughter who is so often noncompliant and very often unpredictable in her behavior from one day to the next can be demoralizing. I would dread the phone calls and notes from the teachers and the school nurse. I tried to develop a good rapport with various teachers, but it would be extra hard to maintain that good working relationship when Rachel would disrupt the classroom on many days.

By now, Rachel's older siblings were teenagers and actively involved in their various activities. Emy actually took on a strong interest in autism, which may have been an important stimulus for her future career as a researcher in developmental psychology, while Matt was also engaged in music, drama, and hockey. They had great friends, worked hard in school, and ultimately both attended GWU as undergraduates. We in turn tried whatever possible to insulate Matt and Emy from a lot of the chaos and disruption generated by Rachel. By no means were we always successful, but we did the best we could.

By this time we had a fourth child, Daniel, who was making the transition from elementary school to junior high school. Our decision to have a fourth child was a difficult one. Many experts and family advised us that once we had one child with ASD, there was a real risk we could have a second. According to some estimates at that time, the likelihood of having a second child with ASD after already having a child with ASD, was around 10 percent. Quite honestly, it was Ann who had the intense desire to have a fourth, and she pushed her agenda hard. Ann's pregnancy with Dan was an anxiety-filled experience. I will never forget that as soon as Dan was born, Ann felt strongly he did not have ASD. She had the same feeling with Dan as she did with Matt and Emy after they were born. By the way Dan interacted with Ann and molded to her countours, she knew that Dan was very different from Rachel and not on the autism spectrum. She turned out to be correct.

We remained in the Washington, DC, area for more than a decade. For my career, GWU was a great launch pad, and being in DC opened up lots of new opportunities for science policy and advocacy. Our vaccine research group was developing an international reputation for our work on new neglected diseases, with an initial emphasis on hookworm infection and schistosomiasis. The work was fulfilling both intellectually as well as emotionally. We had a unique team of scientists using science to pursue humanitarian goals.

Also during this period I was able help shape the policy framework for the NTDs, launching a new open access journal, *PLOS Neglected Tropical Diseases*, and working with the White House and US Congress to get funds appropriated to provide access to essential NTD medicines for people living in poverty. In addition to developing NTD vaccines and bringing NTDs to the world stage through a concerted program of advocacy, I also started writing for the public and in 2008 published my first single-author book, *Forgotten People, Forgotten Diseases,* which is now in its second edition [5].

My time in Washington was one of the most productive of my career. But that was the good news. The bad news was the horrific cost of housing and living and terrible commuting time in DC. Supporting a family on an academic salary in this region became untenable, and I was commuting more than an hour each way to get to work. And there was still the international travel. I felt that my marriage to Ann was one of "divide and conquer." Ann supported Rachel and the other kids while I tried to build "NTD nation." Our relocation to Washington, DC, was great for me professionally, but financially it might not have been the best move for our family. Just as I had to give up on China to preserve the family, I felt increasingly that I would need to do something drastic about our financial situation in the "Roman Empire." Also, I had aspirations to do something bigger, beyond running an academic department.

A New School of Tropical Medicine in Texas

For years I had wanted to create a new school of tropical medicine that resembled the two schools of its kind in the United Kingdom—the Liverpool School of Tropical Medicine and the London School of Hygiene and Tropical Medicine. Both of these institutions, although founded to serve British colonial and business interests, became powerhouses for making new discoveries in tropical diseases and developing new therapies. As someone who wanted to study tropical diseases since childhood, I had known about both schools since an early age. Even though I was fulfilled professonally at GWU, it wasn't a school of tropical medicine.

In 2010, my lifelong dream came true when Baylor College of Medicine and Texas Children's Hospital invited me to visit Houston to give pediatric grand rounds. After a year of discussions and negotiations, I relocated there to establish the National School of Tropical Medicine at the Texas Medical Center (TMC). The TMC is the world's largest medical center—perhaps the first "medical city" with more than 100,000 employees and 60 institutions. Locating a new National School of Tropical Medicine in the TMC made a lot of sense because of the limitless numbers of potential collaborators and the fact that the school would begin modestly in terms of total faculty so that we could achieve a lot through collaborations.

In terms of actually practicing tropical medicine, Houston itself had many attractive features, given its enormous population as the fourth-largest city in the United States and the fact that it was a gateway city to so many immigrants from Latin America and all around the world. Today Houston is considered the most diverse American city and one of the largest immigrant hubs for people coming from Nigeria, India, China, Bangladesh, and Vietnam—really over the developing world. Moreover, the city is booming as a result of the influx of northerners like the Hotez family fleeing economic oppression in expensive urban centers. As I often say, Houston is "hot, flat, and cheap," a term modified from a book on Texas written by *Texas Monthly* senior editor Erica Grieder, titled *Big, Hot, Cheap, and Right* [6].

Another attraction was the generosity of the TMC institutions, especially Texas Children's Hospital and Baylor College of Medicine. These two powerhouses combined resources to establish the National School of Tropical Medicine (NSTM) as a joint venture. On the research side, I was able not only to move our vaccine development operation in its entirety, but also to use the opportunity to expand our portfolio of neglected disease vaccines. In parallel with setting up the NSTM, we also created a unique Texas Children's Hospital Center for Vaccine Development. Essentially, we went from working to develop two vaccines to more than a half-dozen vaccines targeting NTDs such as Chagas disease, leishmaniasis, and onchocerciasis, devastating diseases of the poor that cause severe heart disease, disfiguring ulcers, and blindness, respectively.

To make this happen, my long-standing colleague from GWU, Dr. Maria Elena Bottazzi (who also served as my vice chair for microbiology) and I arranged to move more than a dozen GWU scientists to Houston. The relocation, while daunting, was not as difficult as you might imagine. Our young scientists soon found Houston quite desirable as they left small, crowded condos and 90-minute Washington, DC, commutes to build brand-new yet modestly priced four- and five-bedroom houses in the Houston suburbs of Sugarland, Pearland, and Missouri City to create a better life for themselves and their families.

But there is another side of Houston and Texas, characterized by mostly hidden poverty and disease. Shortly after moving to the city, we determined that tropical diseases are widespread and not linked solely to immigration. Instead, we found a high level of transmission of tropical ailments such as, among others, Chagas disease and Zika virus infection within the state of Texas. We're still working to understand the factors responsible for tropical disease transmission, but so far it looks as if poverty, human migrations, and climate change are important factors. For those reasons, we could study tropical diseases without leaving the United States or even Texas itself. Another interesting finding was that the 20 wealthiest economies (the G20 group) actually account for the greatest number of the world's NTDs, but it is only the poor people who contract these diseases in such prosperous nations. I gave the name "blue marble health" to this finding, which became the subject for my second book [7]. The "blue marble" term refers to the iconic picture of Earth taken by Apollo astronauts during the 1970s.

One concern I had about moving to Houston and leaving the Roman Empire was whether I could maintain my national presence in Texas. But the irony was that just a few years after moving, Ebola arrived in Dallas and Zika virus infection emerged in South Texas. Then there are the potential health issues following the Houston and Beaumont floods associated with Hurricane Harvey. I found myself becoming a national spokesperson for these diseases, with some interesting TV appearances on CNN, Bloomberg, MSNBC, Fox News, and even one bit on the Jon Stewart Show on Comedy Central. Things I could never have predicted!

By this time, our older daughter, Emy, having obtained her PhD in developmental psychology, was living with her new husband Yan and teaching and working at the City University of New York. Matt moved in with us for a time but then struck off for Tucson, Arizona, to work in library science, play music, and live with Brooke, his fiancée (now wife), a doctoral student in English. Daniel became a successful petroleum engineering undergraduate at the University of Oklahoma. All of the kids wound up doing interesting things. But we still had Rachel with us. By now she was an adult with special needs, and her high school years in the Houston Independent Schools were perhaps the rockiest ones yet. A new set of challenges loomed.

· 6 ·

The British Invasion

In the years following the *Lancet* publication of the 1998 Wakefield et al. paper, vaccination rates declined in the United Kingdom and in some countries on the European continent. Measles outbreaks ensued, initially in Europe and then the United States, and are continuing to this day. In the first half of 2017 alone, the Twin Cities of Minneapolis–St. Paul experienced an outbreak of 79 cases among an unvaccinated group of Somali immigrants, with numerous hospitalizations, while Italy reported more than 3,300 cases and 2 deaths. During the year of 2016 and first half of 2017, Romania reported almost 7,500 measles cases and 31 deaths, while other European countries had at least 100 cases or more [1].

Perhaps more than other childhood illness, measles is one of the best indicators for drops in vaccine use among a population. One reason for this observation is that measles is so highly contagious—in fact it is one of the most transmissible infectious agents of humans. We often use the term "reproductive number" (R_0) to indicate how contagious a pathogen is, also known as "transmissibility." For example Ebola virus infection, which in fact is not very contagious unless you are handling the body fluids of someone who recently died of Ebola or who is in the advanced stages of the disease—such as in the case of the two intensive care unit nurses in Dallas, Texas, who took care of Thomas Duncan as he became severely ill in the United States after contracting Ebola in Liberia—has an R_0 of between 1 and 2 (alternative estimates suggest between 1 and 3, or 1 and 4). This value represents the number of people likely to become infected after contact with an Ebola patient. The Ebola R_0 is regarded as relatively low, and this is an important reason why it was possible to contain the virus infection in Guinea, Liberia, and Sierra Leone, even without a vaccine in hand. Rather, international assistance to bolster the health systems of those countries, provided in part by the US military, was sufficient to prevent an epidemic. In contrast, smallpox has an R_0 that ranges between 5 and 7. For such a highly contagious virus, only strategically conducted vaccination programs can be expected to effectively control a smallpox epidemic. Such was the triumph of Dr. D. A. Henderson and his associates. Generally speaking, infectious pathogens with really high R_0 values are best contained through vaccination.

Measles has an R_0 in the 12 to 18 range. This incredibly high number means that we need not only widespread measles vaccine coverage to halt epidemics, but in addition we must maintain our vigilance so that vaccine coverage exceeds 90 to 95 percent. It also means that once this percentage sharply declines, we should expect measles outbreaks. Today, we have seen such big drops and resulting measles epidemics as a result of war and ISIS occupations in Syria and Iraq, or the Taliban threatening vaccinators in Afghanistan. Sadly, we have just seen how an effective anti-vaccine movement that spreads false information about MMR vaccine and autism in the United Kingdom and then Europe has also precipitated a steep decline. Starting in the early years of the 2000s, British-style anti-vaccine sentiments began spreading to the United States, causing small measles outbreaks that ultimately led to larger ones in Texas (2013), California (2014–15), and Minnesota (2017).

Measles Eradication in the United States

Dr. John Enders is not a household name, but he is one of the great heroes of biomedical science and should be better known. In 1897, Enders was born in West Hartford, Connecticut, which also happens to be my hometown. His father was a wealthy CEO of a Hartford-based insurance company and made a large fortune that was bequeathed to his son. John Enders began as an English major at Yale, before switching to science and obtaining his PhD in bacteriology and immunology from Harvard in his early 30s. During this period, he worked in the department headed by the great Hans Zinsser, himself one of the early pioneers of microbiology [2]. Enders moved to the faculty of Boston Children's Hospital in 1946 to establish an infectious diseases laboratory, where he developed new cell line technologies for cultivating viruses, including the polio virus, which enabled the subsequent development of the killed and live vaccines spearheaded by Drs. Jonas Salk and Albert Sabin, respectively. In fact, the only Nobel Prize ever awarded for work on polio was for this discovery. In 1954, Dr. Enders and his associates Drs. Thomas H. Weller and Fred C. Robbins received the Nobel Prize in Physiology or Medicine [2]. Subsequently, Enders, together with Drs. Tom Peebles and Sam Katz, then applied similar technologies to cultivating the measles virus, leading to the development of the first measles vaccine, arguably one of the most important discoveries of the twentieth century. I got to know Sam Katz when he became chair of pediatrics at Duke University, and we remain in contact. I consider Sam one of our field's most distinguished elder statesmen and an eloquent spokesman about the importance of vaccines.

The licensed measles vaccine first became available in the United States in 1963, and then, just as had occurred with invasive Hib disease, measles cases, hospitalizations, and deaths also began to decline precipitously (fig. 4) [3–5]. Some estimates indicate that during the prevaccine era the United States suffered from massive measles epidemics every two or three years, usually in late winter or early spring [3–5]. Such epidemics exacted a devastating toll, including millions of measles cases that resulted in 500 deaths, 4,000 cases of measles encephalitis or SSPE (subacute sclerosing panencephalitis), and 50,000 hospitalizations annually [3–5]. It is important to note that in addition to being highly transmissible, measles is a very bad disease and causes serious illness that can lead to severe pneumonia and encephalitis (brain inflammation). This point is especially significant because the anti-vaccine groups often allege that measles is a mild illness, merely associated with a rash for a few days. In fact, the anti-vaccine lobby has targeted me for my comments and posted a meme and accompanying video on YouTube calling me "The Boy Who Cried Wolf" [6]. Nothing could be further from the truth.

Ultimately, the measles vaccine was coformulated together with new vaccines for mumps and rubella in order to create the MMR vaccine in use today. Dr. Stanley Plotkin, then at the Wistar Institute in Philadelphia, was instrumental in developing the rubella vaccine component, while Dr. Maurice Hilleman at Merck & Co. developed both the mumps vaccine and then the MMR vaccine. Hilleman's efforts are nicely described in a wonderful book written by Dr. Paul Offit at Chil-

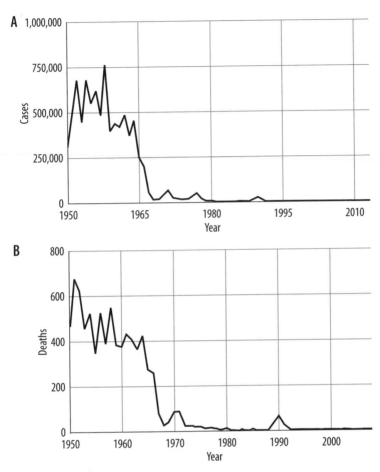

FIGURE 4. Decline in US measles cases (A) and deaths (B) since 1950.

Source: Hotez PJ (2016). Texas and its measles epidemics. PLOS Med 13(10): e1002153, https://doi.org/10.1371/journal.pmed.1002153.

dren's Hospital of Philadelphia, which also highlights the more colorful parts of his character [7]. Hilleman had a masterful command of the English language and was one of the smartest and most entertaining individuals I have ever known. Previously, when I was president of the Sabin Vaccine Institute, we would meet annually at our gold medal ceremony (Hilleman was himself a gold medal awardee), which we typically hosted somewhere in the Baltimore–Washington, DC area.

The current US government guidelines recommend vaccination against measles twice, first between the ages of 12 and 15 months, and then a follow-up with a second dose at four to six years of age, approximately the time of entry into the school system. These ages are important because it means that infants less than 12 months of age are always highly susceptible to measles virus infection. It also means that if measles virus is circulating in a community, parents have to be careful about whether and where to take their infant outside the home. But by the 1980s, measles was near elimination in the United States, and by 2000, there was no longer any sustained measles transmission [8]. The elimination of measles throughout the country was considered one of our nation's most important public health triumphs.

Nonmedical Exemptions and the
Rise of Measles in California

Unfortunately, America's victory over measles in 2000 did not last very long, owing to a rising tide of parents refusing to vaccinate their children. In 2008, 64 cases of measles were reported in several different states, of which 63 were unvaccinated or had an unknown vaccination status. These numbers included 21 children, of whom 14 had been exempted out of vaccines for philosophical or religious beliefs [9].

Today there are almost 20 states that allow nonmedical exemptions, also known as "philosophical exemptions"—exemptions for "personal or moral beliefs"—from school immunization requirements [10]. Of these states, Texas is the largest in terms of population, followed by Pennsylvania, Ohio, Michigan, Washington, and Arizona. In addition, most states, with the exception of California, Mississippi, and West Virginia, allow vaccine exemptions for reasons of religion, although religious exemptions should be uncommon given that the vast majority of the world's religions permit and even enthusiastically support vaccines and vaccinations.

In a recent analysis I conducted in collaboration with Jackie Olive, a Baylor medical student; Ashish Damania, a Baylor staff scientist; and Dr. Melissa Nolan from our faculty, we found a steep rise in nonmedical exemptions since 2009 for most of the 18 states allowing nonmedical exemptions. Moreover, certain US urban areas in these states have especially large numbers of people with nonmedical exemptions, and those likely represent cities at high risk for measles outbreaks. In no particular order they include Detroit, Michigan; Salt Lake City, Utah; Seattle, Washington; Phoenix, Arizona; Portland, Oregon; Boise, Idaho; and Austin, Plano, and other cities in Texas. We're starting to look into the socioeconomic factors underlying the vulnerabilities of these cities.

Not long ago, the state of California was the largest state in the nation allowing both philosophical and religious exemptions to vaccines. However, all of that changed beginning in 2016, when California passed Senate Bill No. 277 (SB 277), which effectively closed the loophole on these nonmedical exemptions. How this happened is an interesting story and one that was tracked recently by Dr. Saad Omer, a professor at Emory University and a vaccine policy expert, together with Dr. Daniel Salmon from the Institute for Vaccine Safety at Johns Hopkins Bloomberg School of Public Health, along with their colleagues [11].

In a paper published in the journal *Vaccine*, the Omer-

Salmon group reported on the impact of philosophical belief exemptions from more than 6,000 public and private California elementary schools. They found that starting in the 1990s and continuing until 2009, the average nonmedical exemption rate increased almost 10 percent annually. Private schools typically showed the sharpest rise. For example, in California private schools the philosophical exemption rate more than doubled between 1994 and 2001, and then almost doubled again by 2009 [11]. Looking at the growth of philosophical exemptions over time in California, especially among private schools, things appeared to really take off in the years immediately following the *Lancet*'s publication of Andrew Wakefield's paper in 1998. This finding does not prove cause and effect, and there certainly could be other factors in play, but to me it suggests that the alleged but spurious links between MMR and autism contributed significantly to the rise in nonmedical exemptions. Did the United Kingdom export its anti-vaccine culture to California? I believe that this is possible, and it is why I titled this chapter "The British Invasion," alluding to a much nicer one in the early 1960s, when we were "invaded" by the Beatles, the Kinks, the Animals, and the Rolling Stones, among others.

In some areas of California such as the North Coast (which includes the Pacific coastal region between Oregon and San Francisco) and Superior California (Sacramento area), the Omer-Salmon group reported that between 5 and 6 percent of elementary school children were philosophically exempted from vaccinations by their parents in the years between 2000 and 2009. Such numbers are significant because we can anticipate measles outbreaks as vaccine coverage drops below 90 to 95 percent. They further found that exemption rates in Los Angeles and Orange Counties, and the San Francisco area were also high. Overall, the researchers found that philosophical exemptions were higher in schools where the population was more likely to be financially comfortable or wealthy and college-educated [11]. A subsequent study found that kindergartens with annual tuitions that exceeded $10,000 were more than twice as likely to have high percentages of their children exempted from vaccines for philosophical reasons, relative to low-tuition kindergartens [12].

I find the demographics of philosophical exemptions especially interesting, because they suggest that parents exempting their kids out of vaccinations are doing so by choice rather than circumstance. Indeed, this has been my experience with much of the anti-vaccine community in the United States. Parents with anti-vaccine leanings often live in wealthier communities and have the education and means to actively search the Internet and follow one or more of the many anti-vaccine websites that are out there. Well-off parents also have in place the social networking to disseminate their findings, as well as the means and leisure time to organize meetings and rallies. They also have the connections and means to lobby local elected leaders and state legislatures.

The rising tide of nonmedical exemptions for philosophical objections created a perfect set-up for measles epidemics to emerge in the state of California. Beginning in the second decade of the 2000s, a major outbreak ensued. According to the CDC, it began in December 2014 with an 11-year-old unvaccinated child who was hospitalized with measles following a visit to a Disney theme park in Orange County, and at least six others who also contracted measles following a Disney visit between December 17 and 20. By early February, the CDC reported in its *Morbidity and Mortality Weekly Reports* (*MMWR*) that

125 measles cases were confirmed, of which more than one-third had visited Disney theme parks and another one-third were secondary cases, meaning that they were close contacts of the individuals who acquired measles at Disney [13].

Tragically, almost one-half of the measles cases occurred among unvaccinated children, including those under the age of one, who were too young to receive their first dose of measles vaccine. In addition, at least 28 measles patients were "intentionally unvaccinated," meaning they deliberately did not receive their measles vaccine because of philosophical beliefs [13]. Many of the unvaccinated individuals were children and teenagers. In addition, another large group had an unknown or undocumented vaccination status. Altogether in the large California measles outbreak of 2014–15 only 11 individuals were known to have received at least one dose of the measles vaccine [13]. The epidemic then spread to Marin County, California, an affluent northern suburb of San Francisco [14].

The 2014–15 California measles epidemic was a reminder about the seriousness of the disease: approximately 20 percent of the cases required hospitalization [13]. The epidemic also illustrated how fragile our public health infrastructure actually is in terms of measles control. The source of the measles was not established, but molecular typing of the virus revealed it was similar or identical to a virus strain that had caused an outbreak in the Philippines. Presumably, just a single individual or perhaps family infected with measles coming into the United States from the Philippines could trigger a significant outbreak among an unvaccinated population, putting many in the hospital [13]. The Disneyland and Marin County measles outbreaks generated a fair bit of finger pointing, and blame was passed around widely. On the popular *Daily Show*, comedian-anchor

Jon Stewart attributed the epidemic to "science-denying, affluent, California liberals" [14], which in my opinion may actually bear some truth.

If there was any silver lining to the California measles outbreak, it's that it woke up the California State Legislature. The
California Senate shut the door by passing SB 277, thereby elim-
inating nonmedical exemptions from both public and private
schools. The resulting impact was immediate and impressive,
as vaccine coverage rates in California increased almost immediately beginning in 2016 when the law went into effect. However, a clause in SB 277 also stated that children who had already obtained nonmedical exemptions prior to the year 2016
could be "grandfathered" in until they reach seventh grade,
so that some exemptions are expected to continue until the
year 2022 [15]. Moreover, in a 2017 op-ed piece, Paul Offit expressed concern that some health-care providers might allow
medical exemptions even in the absence of a true medical in-
dication [16], while in *JAMA Pediatrics* a distinguished group
of investigators suggested that simply shutting down nonmedical exemptions in state legislatures may not be adequate, additional policies in the areas of enforcement, reimbursement for
health-care providers who counsel vaccine-reluctant parents,
and other policy measures may be needed [17]. Still another
concern is the finding by Dr. James Cherry and his colleagues
at UCLA who found that the dreaded delayed and long-term
measles complication known as SSPE is much higher among
California children than previously realized [18]. SSPE is a
progressive and devastating neurologic condition that leads
to coma or death. All this means that even with passage of SB
277, California measles may still be with us at least for the next
few years.

Moving the Problem to Minnesota

As California closed its nonmedical exemptions and slowly climbed out of its measles debacle, a new problem was discovered among the closely knit Somali community in the Minneapolis–St. Paul urban areas of Minnesota. The first wave of Somali immigrants came to the area in the 1980s, but the influx picked up steam after civil wars in Somalia during the 1990s. It's estimated that the Somali community numbers around 25,000 in the Twin Cities.

Minnesota is another large US state that allows philosophical exemptions for vaccines. Among the Somali community, vaccination rates dropped to just over 40 percent in 2014, from over 90 percent a decade before, sparking a substantial local measles outbreak. According to Lena Sun, a *Washington Post* investigative reporter who tracks the American anti-vaccine movement, during this period of decreasing immunization rates Andrew Wakefield had left the United Kingdom in order to relocate near Austin, Texas, but he also visited with the Somali community on at least three occasions in order to speak with Somali families with children on the autism spectrum [19]. As immunization rates and vaccination coverage dropped, a measles outbreak was predictable, especially given that the Minneapolis–St. Paul area receives and sustains continuous waves of immigrants from Somalia, a war-torn area where measles is still widespread. Right on cue, a very large measles outbreak began in April 2017, which as of July resulted in more than 79 cases, just about all of them in children under the age of 10 years and occurring overwhelmingly in non-vaccinated children. At least 21 children were hospitalized.

Vaccination rates among the Somali community showed major reductions beginning around 2008, when children on the autism spectrum began participating in preschool programs [19]. Lena Sun reports how anti-vaccine groups began meeting with the Somali community and helped to promote a significant drop in vaccination rates. At a parent meeting in 2011 that featured Wakefield, an armed guard allegedly barred public health officials and reporters from attending the gathering. Sun quotes Wakefield in her May 5, 2017, article in the *Washington Post*: "'The Somalis had decided themselves that they were particularly concerned,' Wakefield said last week. 'I was responding to that.' He maintained that he bears no fault for what is happening within the community. 'I don't feel responsible at all,' he said" [19]. As of this writing, the Minnesota measles epidemic is finally winding down after lasting for several months.

In both California and Minnesota, we can see the same paradigm: dramatic falls in vaccine coverage rates, especially for MMR, followed by a large measles outbreak ignited by immigration to the United States from a known measles-endemic country—possibly the Philippines in the case of California and Somalia in the case of Minnesota. Indeed, a 2017 study conducted by the CDC identified 1,789 measles cases in the United States from the years 2001 through 2015, as well as 13 outbreaks with 20 or more cases. It found that 10 of the 13 outbreaks occurred after 2010, mostly among patients who were unvaccinated or had unknown vaccination status [20]. As Lena Sun of the *Washington Post* pointed out in her report on the study, "People who don't get vaccinated are the most likely reason for the steady increase in the rate of measles and major outbreaks in the United States" [21]. Also in 2017, I published a study together with Nathan Lo, an MD-PhD student at Stanford University Medical School, showing how quickly measles epidemics can spread among unvaccinated school-aged populations in the United States. We found that a mere 5 percent decline in vaccine coverage can result in a threefold increase in measles cases, at a cost of over $2 million. And that number does not even take into account the unvaccinated infant siblings not yet old enough to receive their measles vaccine [22].

Texas

As events unfolded in California and Minnesota, a new anti-vaccine battleground emerged in the state of Texas. Today, Texas has among the largest number of philosophical or non-medical exemptions in any state. The Department of State Health Services has been tracking an ominous trend that is now rapidly accelerating. Shown in figure 5 is the dramatic rise of nonmedical vaccine exemptions, which have increased almost 20-fold since 2003, such that more than 50,000 children have parents opting them out of getting vaccinated [3].

A major concern about the rise of vaccine exemptions in Texas is that they are not evenly or homogeneously distributed across the state. Instead we're finding that philosophical exemptions appear to cluster in certain hot spots. For example in Travis County, where Austin is located, we see especially high nonmedical exemption rates. The Denton area is another. Today, in and around Austin there are some private schools where 20, 30, or even 40 percent of the students are not vaccinated [3, 23, 24]. At the pricey Austin Waldorf School, more than 40 percent of the students are unvaccinated [23, 24]. Moreover, these numbers also do not take into account the more than three hundred thousand Texas children being home-schooled.

Practically speaking, the large numbers of children receiving nonmedical exemptions means we're likely to see a situation unfold in the Austin area that is similar to what happened

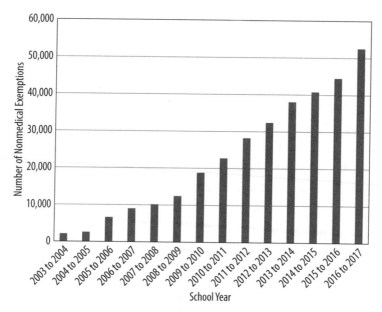

FIGURE 5. Personal belief exemptions in Texas: K–12th-grade students with nonmedical exemptions, 2003–17.

Source: Hotez PJ (2016). Texas and its measles epidemics. PLOS Med 13(10): e1002153, https://doi.org/10.1371/journal.pmed.1002153 (updated to include the 2016–17 school year with data from the Texas Department of State Health Services).

in California in 2015 or in Minnesota in 2017. But I worry things could also get much worse, given the huge number of exemptions and the rapid acceleration in the rate at which kids are being exempted. At the current tempo, it won't be long before we will approach 100,000 children being exempted, with the greatest concentrations in the Austin area.

So what's going on in Austin and Texas? Several things have happened here to help promote a dramatic increase in anti-vaccine sentiments and activities. Prominent among them is the fact that Andrew Wakefield moved to Austin, where he has promoted a film that he wrote and directed [19, 24]. The movie,

Vaxxed: From Cover-Up to Catastrophe, is a self-described documentary that was released in 2016. It attempts to strongly tie autism to vaccinations, especially the MMR vaccine, but it also alleges a vast conspiracy and cover-up by the CDC to hide its links with pharmaceutical companies. The movie is being shown around the state of Texas.

I tend not to use much salty language in my public remarks, but in order to describe *Vaxxed* I make an exception. In my public lectures, I plainly assert that the movie *Vaxxed* is compelling, convincing, and total bullshit. It is less a movie and more a propaganda device to rally unknowing parents toward the pseudoscience of the anti-vaccine movement. Never have I seen such a blatantly dishonest and exploitative piece of nonsense. The *Vaxxed* director and producer went to great lengths to show ASD children at their worst, with a voice-over telling us vaccines are to blame. Beyond the alleged links between MMR vaccine and autism, a central tenet of the film is that the CDC engaged in a vast and complicated cover-up. Among other claims, the movie argues that a CDC scientist found links between vaccinations and autism in African American boys in a study conducted in 2004, but as a potential whistleblower the scientist was silenced by his superiors. Accordingly, the *Vaxxed* filmmakers specifically targeted some African American communities, including Compton, California, at times bringing along some of the leaders of the Nation of Islam [25]. The targeting of African Americans bears an eerie resemblance to similar anti-vaccine efforts to exploit Somali immigrant populations in Minnesota. In both instances, vulnerable populations are being targeted.

Beginning in 2016, the *Vaxxed* filmmakers began showing the film outside of Texas. It almost premiered at the Tribeca Film Festival in New York, only to be pulled by Robert De Niro, a cofounder of the event, following extensive criticisms from the public health community [26]. Still, there were subsequent screenings in New York and multiple other US cities, and even the launch of a self-described "Vaxxed Bus Tour" through urban areas of Arizona, California, Colorado, and Idaho [27].

In Texas, the *Vaxxed* screenings and Andrew Wakefield's other activities are promoted by a self-described political action committee known as "Texans for Vaccine Choice." As the *Washington Post*'s Lena Sun reports, Texans for Vaccine Choice, steeped in the "rhetoric" of Tea Party language [24], in some ways uses a different approach from the efforts that led to the measles outbreak of 2015 in California. Whereas the California anti-vaccine movement is politically liberal and focused on using natural approaches and ingredients in lieu of vaccines, in Texas the focus is more on choice and individual rights.

According to Sun, Jackie Schlegel, who heads Texans for Vaccine Choice, sums it up this way: "Texans value parental rights. We have a message of liberty. We have a message of choice" [24]. My response to this is that the anti-vaccine groups in Texas want it both ways. Imagine that you are a young parent living in the Austin area with an infant not yet old enough to receive its measles vaccine. Wouldn't you be concerned about going into public places with your baby? Wouldn't you think twice about going to a store, church, a new parent support group, even the public library? Texans for Vaccine Choice has effectively stripped civil liberties away from thousands of parents with young children.

Overall, Texans for Vaccine Choice has been an effective anti-vaccine lobby and an important reason I believe non-medical exemptions are rising rapidly and will soon be off the charts. They are well organized and powerful, arranging screenings of *Vaxxed* across the state, holding rallies and marches in the state capital, and going on social media, while meeting with members of the Texas Legislature to file pieces of legislation that make it easier to opt out of vaccines. What I find especially impressive is their website; just clicking on a tab takes a parent or guardian step by step through the nonmedical exemption process.

In 2013, a megachurch located north of Dallas experienced a measles outbreak in which 21 people contracted the illness. The majority of the church parishioners were not vaccinated, including those who came down with measles, and the church had a reputation for being "vaccine-skeptical" [28]. I'm worried the 2013 outbreak is just a harbinger of future measles epidemics in the state of Texas, which is poised for such events on an unprecedented scale. I'm equally concerned that what happened in California in 2015, Minnesota in 2017, and the imminent future of the state of Texas portends a national crisis resulting from epidemics of measles and other childhood illnesses.

The Mercury Scare

In parallel with the expanded activities of Wakefield and his colleagues, Robert F. Kennedy Jr. stepped up his game in early 2017 by holding a well-publicized Washington, DC, press briefing with Robert De Niro at the National Press Club. The major points of the press conference were to further allege the association of thimerosal and mercury with autism, in addition to making claims that the major multinational vaccine manufacturers have censored or squashed any public discussion regarding vaccines. The briefing was also an opportunity to highlight Kennedy's nonprofit organization, the World Mercury Project, which proposes to end industry practices of adding thimerosal or other mercury-containing substances to vaccines. A month later, Kennedy and others led a rally in Washington, DC, on vaccine safety, which like *Vaxxed*, emphasized CDC-industry conspiracy theories. Both the Wakefield and Kennedy camps heavily play up the conspiracy angle.

The anti-vaccine movements in Texas and later in Minnesota may be reaching a new and unprecedented pitch. They are better organized than ever before. Extending these anti-vaccine activities to major media centers in New York and Washington, DC, may indicate a pivot toward the establishment of a national anti-vaccine movement.

Both Wakefield and Robert Kennedy Jr. also claim they met (separately) with Donald Trump during the election or prior to his inauguration, with RFK Jr. indicating he had been asked to head some type of federal vaccine safety commission. In 2014, Trump put out some tweets on social media suggesting he believed vaccines caused autism. For example, on March 28 he wrote, "Healthy young child goes to doctor, gets pumped with massive shot of many vaccines, doesn't feel good and changes—AUTISM. Many such cases" [29]. He then made an anti-vaccine remark at one of the GOP debates in the fall of 2016 [30].

Such statements led to some media speculation that the anti-vaccine movement was somehow being energized by the Trump election and inauguration in January. On these points I am not so sure. After the meeting with Kennedy, the president's transition team denied that any decision had been made about a federal vaccine commission [31], and to my knowledge the president himself has not made any anti-vaccine statements since his inauguration and while he has been in office so far. It's still unclear whether his past statements have some role in a new national trend against vaccinations in the United States. There is lots of chatter about President Trump serving as an enabler of this American neo-anti-vaccine movement, but I don't feel we have the evidence yet to make such statements.

Reversing Global Goals?

Today's modern anti-vaccine movement began in London in 1998 and then spread to the United States in the early 2000s. But I'm worried that things will not stop there. The *Vaxxed* movie has been shown in Ireland, Germany, and Australia— and even in London, where the movement first began. What are the chances that this anti-vaccine movement will be globalized? This is not easy to assess, but I have concerns. For better or worse, the United States exports its culture and values. From my recent experiences as US Science Envoy in the Obama administration, I know that our research universities train a significant percentage of the technocrats and other leaders of nations abroad. Everyone watches movies made in Hollywood. MTV and our popular music is ubiquitous, as is KFC, McDonald's, Subway, and Taco Bell. By the way, I'm not criticizing—instead, I think it's great—I'm a dedicated consumer of American culture abroad. I started writing a previous book in Tokyo, bringing my laptop to McDonald's every morning for breakfast; and in my role as US Science Envoy in Riyadh, Saudi Arabia, lunch catering from Chez Subway was the norm. I love watching MTV music videos when I'm on the morning treadmill in hotels in London, Berlin, Rabat, São Paulo, Mexico City, or Tunis, which for some reason you cannot get with standard cable in the United States. But I'm worried that as word gets out about the ascendancy of the anti-vaccine movement in Texas, along with the Washington, DC, rallies and press conferences, such trends will also spill over into Asia, Africa, and Latin America.

We are already seeing an abundance of anti-vaccine activities in Europe. In 2016, Dr. Heidi Larson and her colleagues at the London School of Hygiene and Tropical Medicine published indices to measure "vaccine hesitancy." They conducted surveys among more than 65,000 individuals in 67 countries to find that Europe is now a hotbed of anti-vaccine sentiments, and they discovered especially high levels of anti-vaccine opinions and low immunization coverage in nations such as France, Italy, Bosnia and Herzegovina, Croatia, and Russia. For example, more than 40 percent of the participants in the survey in France disagreed with the statement that "vaccines are safe" [32]. Interestingly, like California, higher socioeconomic status groups and those with education were more likely to hold anti-vaccine beliefs, although in Europe there are also key factors that go beyond associations with autism, such as general mistrust of vaccines or not accepting the public health importance of the diseases targeted by vaccinations [8, 20, 32]. Anecdotally I have found similar sentiments in the United States, such as when the anti-vaccine groups claim I'm exaggerating the medical and public health consequences of measles epidemics. Despite the massive evidence from Global Burden of Disease studies and multiple other peer-reviewed sources showing that prior to Gavi, the Vaccine Alliance and the launch of the UN's Millennial Development Goals, measles ranked among the leading killers globally (almost one million deaths in 1990, for example), they simply don't accept that measles is a killer of children.

Ultimately, I'm worried that the anti-vaccine movement based in the United States and Europe might devolve into reductions in vaccine coverage in areas that are especially vulnerable to measles. My particular concerns are the very large, low- and middle-income countries (LMICs) such as Brazil,

Russia, India, China, and South Africa, as well as Bangladesh, Nigeria, and Indonesia. Given the size, scope, magnitude, and vulnerabilities of these populations, the consequences of reducing vaccine coverage are enormous. If these nations follow the same playbook seen in the United States and some European countries, we could see reversals of vaccine gains, especially among the middle and higher classes. We already have a different sort of vaccine hesitancy in countries such as Pakistan and Afghanistan, because of the activities of the Taliban and other militant religious groups.

Some evidence is already emerging in Brazil and elsewhere that educated parents are altering their vaccine decisions based on information (or misinformation) provided on the Internet [33]. In *Scientific American* in 2017, I wrote that if an American-style anti-vaccine movement starts hitting the massive LMICs, we could witness measles and other childhood infection outbreaks on a scale not seen in decades. We could even see reversals of the Millennial Development Goals to reduce child mortality [34]. For such reasons, the American anti-vaccine movement must become an immediate and leading concern of our major global health organizations such as Gavi, UNICEF, WHO, and the Gates Foundation, among others. We may need an integrated and coordinated response against this faction, lest vaccine coverage rates drop among vulnerable populations in the world's LMICs. If we are to continue achieving successful reductions in childhood diseases and make progress toward the UN's new Sustainable Development Goals, we're going to have to address the American and soon-to-be-global anti-vaccine movements now, and in a substantive way. Business as usual, which for the US government and major international health agencies has meant turning a blind eye, will ensure our failure.

Montrose

Rachel was an 18-year-old adult when we moved to the Montrose neighborhood of Houston in 2011. The Houston Independent School District (HISD) educates special needs adults until they are 21 or even 22 years of age. At the special needs program at Lamar High School, Rachel's behavioral issues continued, including the inflexibility, the avoidance, and an oppositional component. It was noted that she is "friendly" but "literal," rigid, and easily "upset." A strong obsessive-compulsive element evolved, as described in one evaluation: "During class she asks many questions almost [to] the point of obsessing over certain class routines such as breaks." She asked continuously to use the restroom. "When allowed to use the restroom, Rachel will stay in the restroom for long periods of time in which a staff member will have to redirect her back to class." And her behavior retained a strong oppositional component: "During class time, Rachel will refuse to participate in class activities and at times uses foul language."

Lamar High School

Lamar High School tried hard to provide Rachel with an academic program, and she did ultimately receive a high school certificate. To make this happen, Lamar placed her in a very small special needs classroom, which was also attended to by one or two class aides. The focus of the aides and teachers was to do their best to ensure that Rachel finished in-class tasks and assignments. But because of her noncompliance, Rachel did not attend any regular classes at Lamar except for gym and horticulture. She generally refused to do any homework, and if she did attempt an assignment, it was always rushed and half-done, as Rachel insisted that she had "finished" and needed to get back to her TV shows or computer searches. One of our big regrets was never being able to get Rachel to focus on homework or completing other tasks. This inability later proved to become part of her undoing while looking for employment.

For several years the head teacher in Rachel's class was "Coach Johnson," who also served as Lamar's assistant football coach. Coach Johnson was a formidable presence, and we heard that in the past he actually had some NFL tryouts. But he was a gentle giant who really looked after Rachel and helped ensure that she wasn't bullied, which can be a huge problem for teenagers with ASD. Even after high school, Rachel would run into Coach Johnson at Randall's supermarket, where each morning Rachel got her plain bagel (no butter) and Coach Johnson, his coffee. Rachel was proud when Coach Johnson complimented her on her independence and ability to walk more than a half-mile each way to get breakfast. Rachel's other favorite teacher was Ms. Coleman, who bonded well with Rachel and even visited her during the short time in which Rachel had a residential placement outside the home.

While at Lamar, Rachel was required to develop a "visual résumé." In the section titled "Things I Like to Do," it's interesting to see how many of the bullet points relate to travel or independence:

- I enjoy discussing protection of people, animals, and the environment
- I enjoy walking to the store or Subway and using my debit card to make purchases
- I love to practice riding the Metro bus
- On the weekends, I have brunch with family and friends
- I am interested in having more friends and doing more fun things
- I like to review maps of where the Metro goes to find out how to get places
- I have fun going to the zoo and parks
- I want to make money to be able to travel
- I am planning a trip to the Atlanta Aquarium
- I like to go places, riding with my brother who drives now
- I like going to get my hair and nails done
- I've been learning to do chores and cook

Ann and I interpreted this to mean that there was a part of Rachel that, as do many young adults, craves adventure and independence, but maybe she feels trapped by intellectual disabilities.

At Lamar, Rachel met her first real and age-appropriate friend, a girl named Sabrina. Like Rachel, Sabrina was personable and quite vocal, and also on the autism spectrum. Both girls have a strong personality, and each was able to convince the other to share a mutual interest or obsession. For instance, Rachel convinced Sabrina that the Power Rangers were cool, while Sabrina taught Rachel about Ariana Grande, Justin Bieber, and Austin Mahone, as well as other pop music stars. Together they would share outrageous gossip stories about interactions between Miley Cyrus and Justin Bieber, some of which you might find in the *National Enquirer* but many others that were just totally made up. They seem to completely enjoy each other's company and feed off their mutual enthusiasm. Interestingly, before she met Rachel, Sabrina was quite timid about going places on her own and walking around Houston neighborhoods. Rachel was able to help Sabrina achieve some level of independence and walk places. Having said that, Sabrina was also compliant and followed directions, which made it possible for her to have more success at school and get a paid internship, whereas Rachel's opposition and unwillingness to comply largely blocked her. It was a sad moment when Sabrina's father had to relocate to Denver. However, two years later, Rachel and Sabrina still talk on the phone twice a day, starting at 3:00 or 4:00 a.m. (with ASD, both girls wake up in the middle of the night), and they also Skype. Rachel has even flown by herself to Denver on Southwest Airlines, but with a lot of help getting her to and from the airport and the cooperation of some wonderful Southwest flight attendants.

Rachel graduated from her structured high school program in 2014. Her final evaluation at Lamar listed "autism" as a "primary handicapping condition" and "intellectual disability" as her "secondary handicapping condition." She refused to attend graduation because it required waiting in a long line with no access to her TV shows. It also required Rachel to wear a cap and gown, which she also refused. For us, not even being able to commemorate or celebrate Rachel's high school graduation was particularly disappointing.

Houston Community College

Rachel was 21 years old when she finally left Lamar to attend an innovative and very thoughtful special needs program that was organized jointly by the Houston Independent School District and Houston Community College (HCC). It was called the "transition program," and many of the young adults who completed the transition program could then go to the VAST Academy continuing education program. Ann and I felt this offered the best opportunity for Rachel to transition to her new working life as an adult. Unfortunately, she quickly bounced out of the program, owing to her lack of compliance and disruptive behavior. It was around this time that a new obsessive-compulsive behavior—namely, an incessant asking of questions, usually the same question over and over again—began taking over a part of her personality. To ask her questions, Rachel would interrupt the teacher continuously, to the point where it became impossible for the teacher to continue. In one case, it included a teacher who previously knew Rachel at Lamar and liked her, but even she could not manage this new postgraduate Rachel. In addition, the oppositional behavior would continue, and she would use profanity, or try to leave the classroom and spend time in the women's bathroom. Rachel would not do the homework assignments and simply showed no interest in the academic activities required at HCC.

Rachel's refusal or inability to navigate the transition program forced its staff to bounce her back to Lamar High School to complete the year. All of Rachel's teachers were deeply disappointed that Rachel had gone backward. As you can imagine, this setback was devastating for Ann, because it proved that this was the end of the road for Rachel's educational advancement. It meant she would never attend the VAST Academy, which was superb in that it gave students opportunities to transition to internships and then jobs.

A Special Needs Adult

As things were going badly with HCC, we decided to try something different and to place Rachel in a residential setting. Maybe, we thought, it would help "reset" her. The Center (formerly the Center for Mental Retardation) was just a couple of miles from our home and reasonably priced. We could afford it. But Rachel was too disruptive for the level of supervision that the home provides, and then she began stealing or hoarding money and food from fellow residents. In the end, the Center was not really set up for supervision, and she often left without signing out. We were horrified when Rachel walked by herself at night through the streets of Houston, which has its fair share of crime, once showing up at our doorstep at four o'clock in the morning. Soon after, she was asked to leave the Center.

However, Rachel did make a second friend at the Center, whose name is Lee. He's quite a bit older and, unlike Rachel, has a college degree and a master's degree, but he is also on the autism spectrum. He's now a paralegal and an aspiring law student. Even though both are out of the Center now, Lee still comes to the house to help Rachel learn how to use the Houston bus system and even gives her some cooking lessons. One of Rachel's positive facets is that she is able to make and maintain friendships.

Since then, Rachel has lived at home. We had moved to Montrose, an interesting bohemian neighborhood located just three miles from the Texas Medical Center. The main strip is on Westheimer Avenue, which is dotted with many great cafés, yoga studios, restaurants, vintage clothing shops, and tattoo parlors. Montrose has some similarities to a college town, but with a lot more grit and unevenness. And by that I mean literal "unevenness"; the live oak trees push up the sidewalks several feet in the air to produce what some call the "concrete Alps." But these trees that line the residential areas of Montrose are also arranged to produce a glorious canopy effect. Most of the houses themselves are either bungalows or craftsman-style houses. However, with each passing year there are more and more townhomes, like the one we live in. Another great feature of Montrose is its nearby museums and parks. The Rothko Chapel and the Menil Collection are within walking distance of our home. So all in all, Montrose is an interesting and culturally rich, but not too precious neighborhood. It's a place where tattoo artists, chefs, museum curators, shop owners, and some academics mix with the homeless.

It turns out that Montrose suits Rachel quite well. These days, she is out and about in the neighborhood taking long walks in pursuit of her morning bagel or some other food, a sandwich from Subway, or she'll go into Torchy's Tacos, Fuzzy's Tacos, or Yogurt Land. We'll also send her out on errands to various supermarkets, especially HEB (which has free food samples) for laundry detergent, cat food, or other sundry items. Rachel also loves bakeries and will wander into several different ones to gawk at the cakes and report back to Ann in detail about them.

When Rachel was a little girl, she had a tremendous aversion to trying new foods. "I don't like it—I never even tried it," she would say. Yogi Berra couldn't have said it better. Except possibly for french fries, she also had no real understanding of vegetables. One fall day in Cheshire, I remember pushing Rachel in her stroller when the wind was blowing. As a leaf flew past her, she asked, "What's that, a piece of broccoli?" For many years, she would eat fewer than a dozen foods. No fish, some fruit—she likes bananas—and very few vegetables. Left on her own, she still would prefer a steady regimen of fast food and cakes. In Montrose, we try hard to find innovative ways to incentivize Rachel to eat more healthy foods and snacks, but it requires intense vigilance. Reminding her about risks of obesity is sometimes helpful in persuading her to reduce snacking, sweets, and overall food intake. The fact that she walks for much of her day in our neighborhood and enjoys being out and about is a positive development.

Rachel has an intense curiosity about people, and that means she'll strike up conversations with practically anyone she meets on her daily walks and routines. It's been noted that autism in girls is more difficult to diagnose because they often have much greater social skills compared with boys [1, 2]. This feature stems from either inherent or acquired abilities to mask some key autism traits. Another feature about the girls is that they often have significant coexisting conditions, such as obsessive-compulsive disorder (OCD), anxiety disorder, ADHD, or even anorexia [1]. In these cases, the ASD component is often missed. That's a long way of saying that girls diagnosed with OCD, anxiety disorder, ADHD, or anorexia may in fact have underlying autism. Rachel is friendly, verbal, and curious, and she can be very sociable. Once I accompanied Rachel to a local convenience store, where she introduced me to her new friend, Vin, who I believe owns the store and works behind the register. "Dad, this is my friend Vin. Vin is from Vietnam, but he doesn't speak much English."

If Rachel decides to purchase something, often she will simply pull a bunch of single dollar bills out of her purse, open her hand to the store clerk, and say, "Here." Counting money is extremely difficult; simple math is a constant struggle. Fortunately, the merchants of Montrose, mostly immigrants to Houston from just about everywhere, are incredibly honest, earnest, and hard-working, and they have never taken advantage of Rachel.

Morning and evening dog walkers are some of Rachel's favorite inquisition targets. She knows dog breeds in detail and will quiz the owners about their pets. "Is that a German shepherd mix?" "Is it a schnoodle?" She's particularly drawn to people in wheelchairs or with service dogs. "Why are you in a wheelchair?" she'll ask, or "Why do you have a service dog?" or "Why are you on crutches?" But the conversation almost always winds up as a happy or meaningful discussion. Many disabled individuals in our neighborhood are quite lonely and appreciate the genuine human interaction, especially once they figure out that Rachel means no harm. In the beginning, her direct questioning and interrogation of people with obvious disabilities was sometimes cringeworthy for members of our family. We got used to it once we realized the benefits for both Rachel and her newfound friends. Rachel has enormous patience for people with disabilities, and she is an inherently open and nonjudgmental individual. Once you get past the initial awkwardness, people tend to feel comfortable speaking with her.

One of Rachel's favorite neighbors is Karen, an anesthesiologist who lives next door with her family and works at the Texas Medical Center. Aware of Karen's busy schedule, we admonish Rachel not to be too intrusive, but when Rachel started texting constantly, even when Karen was working in the operating room, we had to remove the number from her cell phone. Rachel will go over to Karen's house whenever she can (or is allowed), and she has even become friends with Karen's visiting parents. Another favorite is Paula, who does Rachel's hair once a week. Sadly, Rachel may have gotten Paula fired: Paula had an argument with her boss over the fact that the boss no longer welcomed Rachel into the salon unless she had an appointment. After the boss made some derogatory remarks about Rachel, Paula stood up and defended Rachel's special needs and rights. She was sacked on the spot. Paula is a hero. We of course were upset when we heard the story but were also concerned by how devastating Paula's firing was for Rachel. Rachel felt terrible remorse and cried about it for many weeks afterward. Paula is now working again, but Ann has to drive Rachel to Paula's new salon. Paula also incorporates Rachel into her personal life. If Paula goes out with friends to a restaurant, or with her boyfriend, Kevin, Rachel is sometimes invited. Rachel knows many of Paula's friends, and vice versa. Between Sabrina, Lee, Karen, and Paula, Rachel has created an interesting and diverse network of friends. She's fiercely loyal to them, as are they to her. It's one of the truly positive elements of Rachel's personality.

Rachel has a great capacity for empathy, for both people and animals. She often cries during TV commercials for UNICEF, Save the Children, ASPCA, and PETA. She always wants to help with a financial contribution. Sometimes I hear Rachel telling people that her dad is making vaccines so they can be used by UNICEF—who knows, maybe one day it will happen! It was because of Rachel that we wound up adopting two shelter cats, and each day she gives them food and water. Neither Ann nor I ever considered ourselves "cat persons," but we have grown to like them. As a component of her empathy, Rachel has an interest in diseases and is typically the one who reminds us about receiving her annual flu vaccine in the fall. She was the one who requested the HPV cervical cancer vaccine. She is

curious about different diseases and illnesses, and grateful that
we have so many vaccines available to stop most of the killer
childhood diseases, but she often asks me why I'm not making
a vaccine for this one or that one. I explain that vaccines take
a long time to make and they are hard work, so it's all we can
do to manage the five or six vaccines now under development
at our Texas Children's Hospital Center for Vaccine Development. For Rachel the idea that vaccines could have caused her
autism is absurd. Smart lady!

Sometimes Rachel's sociability and empathy can also get
her into trouble. On at least two occasions, Rachel has invited
homeless adult men into our house. In one instance, the man
actually went upstairs to the second floor and said hello to
Ann; in the other case, I had to ask the man to leave the house,
and he argued with me. Both episodes ended well in terms of
no one getting injured, but we're worried that this type of behavior could turn out badly either for us or for Rachel. Also,
both episodes are distressing reminders that Montrose is in a
city, and there is crime. Rachel is highly vulnerable, and perhaps our current arrangement is not a sustainable long-term
solution. We're going to have to come up with something better or at least more protected.

On Saturdays evenings, Rachel and I sometimes walk to
a restaurant, order from the take-out menu, and then walk
home to have our dinner (we're pictured in fig. 6). Houston
ranks high among the most international cities and largest immigrant hubs in the United States (I joke that no one is actually from Houston—including us), and Montrose is famous
for its variety of restaurants, especially all sorts of international foods. Rachel loves learning about different foods and
has become a lot more adventurous compared with her early
childhood. Currently, one of her favorite TV shows is *Diners,*

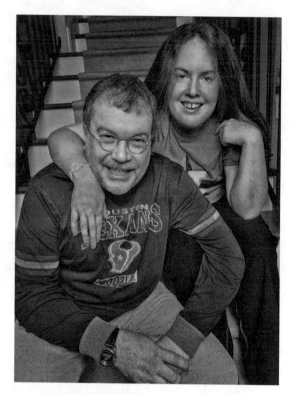

FIGURE 6. Rachel and I at home in 2017.

Photograph by Brian Goldman.

Drive-Ins, and Dives—a show about different low-budget food venues across the country. It's one of the few TV shows we'll actually watch together. During our walks to and from the chosen eatery, we usually talk about all the things she is typically interested in. They include topics related to different animals or travel destinations, and she will even ask me about the diseases I study and our vaccines. She's fascinated by illness.

However, because of her obsessive behavior, in the days prior, she will phone me to remind me about Saturday, and on Saturday itself, she will phone me multiple times, often hourly.

"Dad we're going at 6:15 p.m. on next Saturday, right?" she'll say. "And we're going to Empire Café [a local Montrose diner]?"

"Sure Rach. Wherever you want, sweetie."

Rachel will then rattle off the names of four or five different places, such as Empire Café, but also Brasil Café, Pistolero's, Doc's, El Real, and the list goes on.

"Fine, Rachel, wherever you want."

"We're going at 6:15 p.m.?"

"Yes, Rachel."

"On Saturday?"

"Yes, Rachel."

"6:15 p.m."?

"Yes Rachel, I have to go now, I'm in a meeting."

"OK dad, I love you."

An hour later, the call will be repeated.

If Ann promises Rachel that she can go to a movie on a Tuesday with a friend, about 10 days before, Rachel will start asking Ann whether the event is still happening and when Ann will get money out of the ATM in order to pay for it. She will constantly interrupt conversations and phone calls to ask about the movie, the time, and when Ann will go to the ATM. It's gotten to the point that her questions become almost punishing. Not uncommonly, Rachel will ask the same question four or five times over an hour-long period. We are reluctant to give her things to look forward to because she can be so exhausting and draining.

If thunderstorms are predicted in the weather forecast, Rachel will knock on our bedroom door and our neighbor's door, or phone and text Ann and me continuously to receive reassurance that we won't lose our power or cable: "We're not going to lose our power, are we?" "I don't want to lose our power." And then she'll proceed to repeat this on multiple occasions. Texas can get some impressive lines of thunderstorms, and Rachel has tremendous anxiety about losing power and cable to our house and not having access to TV. She meticulously plans TV watching and viewing specific websites, and the prospect of having that interrupted by power loss is almost more than she can bear. Ann and I are in no position to provide such assurance, but for everyone's peace of mind and to calm Rachel, we often make this promise anyway. Rachel really tests us with her OCD and incessant questions. Ann and I sometimes disagree on how to handle her in this regard. Ann will typically just say "yes" to every question, and I think that just encourages Rachel. I will say "no" or "never," which usually quiets her down, but if both of us are in the house at the same time, between Ann's "yes" and my "no," it makes everybody crazy.

In recent years, Rachel and I have spoken more and more about autism and her ASD, as well as her mental disabilities. She has come to understand that her mental disabilities and negative behaviors have blocked her pathway to employment. Rachel wants a job and wants to earn money, but so far all of our attempts to help her meet her goals have not gone very far. For now, every morning around 4:00 a.m. Rachel Skypes Sabrina. By 7 a.m., Rachel is out walking the neighborhood, headed to Randall's supermarket to buy a bagel. On some days, she's willing to substitute a visit to Dunkin' Donuts, or sometimes on Sunday I'll go with her to the Kolache Factory—kolaches are a Texas specialty: meat or vegetable-filled pastries first introduced by the sizable Czech community that emigrated here in the 1800s. Although her daily routine can be highly caloric, she does a prodigious amount of walking, sometimes five to six miles or more.

She then returns home, heads upstairs to her room, and watches TV or surfs the Internet, and then she's out again before noon to Subway in order to order the same sandwich each day—six-inch tuna, no cheese, with mustard on "hearty Italian." After more conversations with people in the neighborhood or shopkeepers and merchants, it's back to her room, out later for frozen yogurt, then a long nap, and then dinner with the family. Rachel is usually asleep quite early in the evening, but like many with ASD, she has an altered sleep-wake cycle such that she's up for a few hours in the middle of the night on the Internet or watching TV. Rachel often talks to the TV or computer and can be pretty loud and boisterous, at which point Ann or I have to get up and knock on her door, asking her to quiet down.

Right now, we have more questions than answers about Rachel. The current arrangement is working at some level, and Rachel is growing and learning through her daily activities and social interactions. But at the same time, she's not acquiring the skills that will make her employable, and her personality is so strong and oppositional that we are unsure whether her having a job will be an attainable goal. Ann and I are still hopeful, but we feel the windows of opportunity are closing. We've recently gotten connected with Goodwill Industries International, an impressive American nonprofit that has been willing to step in and see if it can help with Rachel. Given that it seems we've exhausted most other options, Goodwill may be our last resort for the foreseeable future. We've become very impressed with Goodwill. The people who work there are committed and friendly, and they have an amazing desire to help people with special needs. Goodwill has arranged a job coach to help Rachel sort clothes, and so far she is sticking with it. We almost don't want to get our hopes up, given Rachel's past record, but right now Goodwill is our last best chance.

We worry a lot, and Ann especially is often up at night thinking about Rachel and her future. We know that we're not alone on this front. Thousands of parents living with adults (or children transitioning to adulthood) who are on the autism spectrum are equally concerned or fretful.

Vaccines Don't Cause Autism

THE SCIENTIFIC EVIDENCE

An important research arm of our National School of Tropical Medicine is an academic research institute known as the Texas Children's Center for Vaccine Development (Texas Children's CVD), a unique organization belonging to a group of so-called product development partnerships (PDPs) that makes vaccines for neglected tropical diseases (NTDs) and other poverty-related neglected diseases. I personally will not make money on our NTD vaccines. My reason for making this statement is that some anti-vaccine groups have alleged otherwise. At least one blogger claims that I make millions of dollars in profit from my vaccines. If only! So far, I've not received a penny; I have no real prospects for financial gain; nor do I seek monetary reward from my vaccines. These vaccines target diseases that afflict the poorest of the poor, and I am an academic professor and dean whose salary comes from Baylor College of Medicine and Baylor University, offset by research grants from government agencies and well-established non-profit private philanthropies. Another prominent anti-vaccine group points out that I hold several patents for our antipoverty vaccines. This is true, but I have taken this measure only to protect the intellectual property (IP) from being blocked by other for-profit organizations or concerns. As an alternative strategy, we do not file IP patents for some of our vaccines because of the expense, especially for foreign filings, but instead simply publish our findings in peer-reviewed biomedical journals so as to get the information out in the public domain.

The Antipoverty Vaccines

Globally there are about 20 product development partnerships, which are nonprofit associations that use industry practices for making drugs, diagnostics, or vaccines for diseases of poverty, including AIDS, malaria, tuberculosis, and the NTDs. One of the better-known ones is the Drugs for Neglected Diseases initiative that makes small-molecule drugs for these conditions. Another is the Medicines for Malaria Venture. Our organization is a vaccine PDP specific for NTDs. Today the NTDs comprise the most common afflictions of people who live in extreme poverty. Indeed, almost every human being affected by poverty is also afflicted with an NTD. Most of the NTDs are chronic and debilitating infections that may actually promote poverty. Because these diseases make people too sick for gainful employment or have the ability to reduce child intelligence and development, or because they adversely affect pregnancy outcome, vaccines that target NTDs are sometimes referred to as "antipoverty vaccines."

Our Texas Children's CVD currently has a portfolio of a half-dozen antipoverty vaccines under development. For example, through support from NIH's National Institute of Allergy and Infectious Diseases we're making vaccines for parasitic worm infections such as schistosomiasis, hookworm infection, and onchocerciasis (river blindness)—three diseases that together infect 750 million people in the poorest parts of the world, including Asia, Africa, and Latin America. In addition, through US Department of Defense funding, we're making a vaccine for cutaneous leishmaniasis, also known as "Aleppo evil," because it disfigures children and adults living in the Middle East, North Africa, and Central Asia, where hundreds of thousands of people living in war zones are being infected by the *Leishmania* protozoan parasite through sand fly bites. Leishmaniasis is also a major threat to US troops deployed to Afghanistan and Middle Eastern conflict zones. We're especially proud to support the US military. On that front, we're also helping in the development of new vaccines for emerging mosquito-transmitted viruses, such as West Nile virus infection, while also embarking on coronavirus vaccines for SARS and MERS, as part of a consortium of collaborators.

Finally, through support of the Carlos Slim Foundation, Kleberg Foundation, the Japan Global Health and Innovation Technology Fund, and the Southwest Electronic Energy Medical Research Institute, we're also developing a new vaccine for Chagas disease, another parasitic protozoan infection, but transmitted by triatomines ("kissing bugs"), that affects almost 10 million people in the poorest parts of Latin America. Today, Chagas disease is one of the leading causes of severe heart disease among the poor in the Western Hemisphere. Recently, scientists at our National School of Tropical Medicine also found a significant level of Chagas disease transmission within the state of Texas. In fact, we've found that NTDs and other poverty-related neglected diseases are widespread as a result of local transmission, especially among the poor.

I often say that our Texas Children's CVD makes the vaccines that the major multinational pharmaceuticals cannot develop because the diseases they target exclusively affect people living in extreme poverty. There is little or no financial remuneration for such vaccines, so that publicly owned companies would not be able to make money for their shareholders if they took on the vaccines listed in our portfolio. Instead, we take the leadership in developing antipoverty vaccines.

The "Vaccines Don't Cause Autism" Papers

The false accusation that vaccines could be responsible for an "autism epidemic," as the anti-vaccine groups allege, is abhorrent to me because the vaccine-autism link has no scientific basis. Many of the statements and materials put forward by the anti-vaccine communities, including the content of the *Vaxxed* movie and public statements by leaders of anti-vaccine groups, are either false or some pseudoscience half-truth. The latter are perhaps the most interesting, because the anti-vaccine groups often attempt to justify their assertions by using selected pieces of scientific facts, or "factoids," strung together in ways to make their assertions seem plausible. Oftentimes the anti-vaccine proponents address autism and vaccines by trying to make the facts fit their spurious hypotheses, rather than using the scientific method of building the hypothesis around the facts. They have a foregone conclusion and will assemble a series of unrelated pieces and then connect them in ways that were never intended. In so doing, they build a story that at first glance seems as if it might be plausible, but in the end it does not hold up in the face of a serious investigation or large study.

As the anti-vaccine movement gained renewed strength, especially in the United States, I took it upon myself to launch a small, modest counteroffensive. I began by assembling the scientific literature showing that vaccines don't cause autism and also summarizing the latest findings about the neurobiology of autism and explaining why it's not even plausible for vaccines to cause autism. My intention was to release this information on free and publicly accessible websites. My efforts were modest because I had no backing of any particular organization or the US government. I was especially saddened that our nation's public health leaders are so silent about promoting vaccines and vaccination and mostly unwilling to publicly go up against the anti-vaccine community. It's curious to note that such silence has pretty much transcended presidential administrations over the past two decades. Instead, many times I find that efforts to challenge the anti-vaccine movement have included just myself and a few colleagues, our laptops, and sometimes just a few sympathetic e-mails or statements on social media.

My initial efforts resulted in two articles I published as blogs. The first attempted to summarize recent papers from major and high-impact biomedical journals that refute links to autism, while the second tried to point out why autism is a genetic and epigenetic set of conditions that are well under way during prenatal development—way before an infant ever receives a vaccine. This chapter outlines the findings I presented in that first report, a piece I wrote for *PLOS* titled "The 'Why Vaccines Don't Cause Autism' Papers" [1]. The scientific underpinnings of my second contention, that autism develops before birth, is the subject of the next chapter.

A major goal of my *PLOS* blog, which was first published in January 2017, was not to reinvent the wheel in terms of other articles already published on the subject, but to update an extraordinary document put out by the American Academy of Pediatrics (AAP). AAP is an important organization of more than 60,000 pediatricians who are committed to the health of children, adolescents, and even young adults. It is an independent organization, not connected to the US government, but it is instrumental in shaping policies and clinical guidelines for

America's children. In 2013, AAP put out on its website a document of 21 pages listing and summarizing the major scientific papers firmly showing that there is no link between vaccines and autism [2]. The studies specifically show that there are no links between MMR vaccine and autism, and none between thimerosal and autism. In addition to looking at MMR vaccine and thimerosal, the AAP lists scientific papers that also show no links between multiple vaccines given at once and autism. Finally, while some vaccines given to infants can cause a temporary fever, and fever from any cause can result in seizures ("febrile seizures" are overwhelmingly self-limited), the AAP document shows that these side effects are also not linked to autism [2].

Lack of Any Association between MMR Vaccine and Autism

In the years immediately following the publication of the Wakefield et al. paper in the *Lancet*, a number of large studies were conducted to try to confirm or refute a link between MMR vaccine and autism. For example, in 2002 in the *New England Journal of Medicine*, a large Danish study reported on over 500,000 children who had received the MMR vaccine, representing approximately two million patient years (the sum of individual units of time that the subjects in the study population have been exposed to or at risk from the conditions of interest). The retrospective cohort study looked at children born in Denmark between 1991 and 1998, based on the Danish Civil Registration System, with their autism status determined by the Danish Psychiatric Central Register [3]. A retrospective (or historic) cohort study is one of the standard inquiries used by epidemiologists or scientists who study diseases among large populations. It examines a group (cohort) of people with a common exposure to a specific agent, in this case, the MMR vaccine. The study collects information about the cohort from past medical records, looking at how the exposure affected the development of an illness or disease, in this case, autism. Altogether, there were more than 700 children with a diagnosis either of autistic disorder or autistic spectrum disorder. There was no difference in autism rates between the 440,655 children who got the MMR vaccine compared with the 96,648 children who did not get vaccinated [3]. The major finding of the study was that it "provides strong evidence against the hypothesis that MMR vaccination causes autism." In addition, the authors found that there was no "temporal clustering" of autism cases following immunization [3].

Two years later, in 2004, a group led by scientists at the London School of Hygiene and Tropical Medicine reported the results of a case-control study in the *Lancet*. A case-control study is a second and also standard type of epidemiological investigation. Such studies look at the cases, referring to subjects who have the condition or illness, in this case autism, and compare them with controls without autism. In so doing, the epidemiologist can look at whether there are differences between these two groups in terms of whether or not they have received a specific intervention, such as a vaccine. Specifically, the London group looked at almost 1,300 kids with autism (or pervasive developmental disorder) with a median age of 5.4 years and compared them with almost 4,500 controls, with a median age of 4.9 years. Using a UK General Practice Database, they found there was no autism association with MMR vaccination [4].

In yet another experimental study, in 2006, scientists and pediatricians from McGill University and Montreal Children's Hospital reported that, contrary to findings of the 1998 paper in the *Lancet* (alleging that measles replicates in the gastro-intestinal tract), there is no evidence of persisting measles virus from MMR-vaccinated children with autism [5]. Specifically, the McGill group looked at the white cells found in blood (peripheral blood mononuclear cells) from more than 50 children with ASD and 34 children who were developmentally normal, and conducted up to six polymerase chain reactions (PCRs) looking at two different measles virus genes. PCR is the most sensitive method known to detect the presence of a virus (actually, the virus genome). The group found no evidence of detectable measles virus in either the autism cases or controls and also found there was no difference between these two groups in blood tests that measure the levels of measles antibodies [5].

Each of the papers highlighted above was also cited in the 2013 AAP document [2]. Since that publication, there have been at least three very large, even massive, studies showing there is no link between the MMR vaccine and autism [6–8]. In 2015, the Lewin Group, a Washington, DC–area health-care consulting firm, together with the Drexel (University) Autism Institute in Philadelphia, conducted a retrospective cohort study of 95,727 children who had older siblings [6]. The researchers relied on a database from a large, private insurer US health plan, known as the Optum Research Database, that includes tens of millions of "both commercially insured individuals and Medicare managed care enrollees." The database also collects data from across the United States and is not confined to a single geographic area. Their study, published in *JAMA* (*Journal of the American Medical Association*), looked at almost 100,000 children, including approximately 1,000 children with autism. In addition, 1,929 children had an older sibling with autism. The MMR vaccination rate among the children with autism or their siblings was high. Approximately 84 percent received at least one dose by the age of two years, and 92 percent by the age of five. Altogether it was found that receipt of the MMR vaccine was not linked to autism, and this was true whether or not the children had an older sibling with autism [6]. This latter finding is important, since it suggests that MMR vaccine is not triggering autism, even among children who may be at higher risk because they are genetically related to a child with autism [6]. Such a finding is especially relevant given that a common assertion made by anti-vaccine groups is that only the children at risk of autism are the ones likely to actually develop autism as a result of vaccination. The *JAMA* study clearly refutes such speculation.

Also in 2015, a Japanese group conducted a case-control study among children born between the years 1986 and 1992 [7]. They studied 189 children diagnosed with ASD at the Yokohama Psychodevelopmental Clinic in the Kaino area of Japan, together with more than 200 controls matched for age and sex. The Japanese scientists found no differences in MMR vaccinations between these two groups, and also that MMR vaccinations were not associated with increased risk of autism. Their conclusion was that "MMR vaccination . . . did not elevate the risk of ASD onset in this Japanese population," and "[t]herefore, there is no need to avoid these vaccinations due to concern of inducing ASD." Instead they conclude appropriately, "We believe it is necessary to explore genetic factors as well as conduct research that accounts for environmental factors in order to elucidate the pathology of ASD. These may lead to early diagnosis of ASD or the development of a biomarker to identify high-risk groups, which may, in turn, contribute to improved quality of life for ASD patients and their families." [7] In my view, this is a key point: because so much effort has now been invested in showing that vaccines don't cause autism, we're becoming distracted from looking at the true genetic and environmental causes.

Finally, in 2014 a group at the University of Sydney in Australia conducted a large data analysis, known as a systematic review or meta-analysis of 10 published studies, including five case-control studies and five cohort studies [8]. Such systematic reviews are useful in looking at the aggregate of major scientific publications in a given field and sometimes allow one to analyze data from a million children or more. Their search of PubMed and other databases identified more than 1,000 papers, most of which did not meet the criteria for inclusion in the meta-analysis. To meet the criteria, the studies had to be either a retrospective or prospective cohort study or a case-control study, such as those highlighted above. Altogether, they identified 10 studies involving more than 1.2 million children, with two studies looking specifically at the MMR vaccine, two at cumulative mercury dosage, and one at thimerosal exposure [8]. Once again there was no association between multiple MMR vaccines (or thimerosal-containing vaccines) and the development of autism or ASD.

Together the studies highlighted here provide overwhelming evidence that there is no link between MMR vaccination and autism or ASD. They represent large and well-documented studies conducted in the United States, Europe, and Japan.

Lack of Any Association between Thimerosal and Autism

A second major factor often implicated in causing autism is thimerosal, which was previously contained in many US vaccines [9] but has since been taken out except for some multi-dose pediatric flu vaccines. But even for flu, there are now pediatric vaccines currently in use in the United States that also do not contain thimerosal [10]. As pointed out previously, the US Food and Drug Administration never found evidence that thimerosal in pediatric vaccines caused harm, but nevertheless the agency recommended its removal as an overall precaution and desirability of reducing any type of childhood mercury exposure. Because thimerosal is mostly used in multi-dose vials to prevent bacterial contamination, the FDA worked with the vaccine manufacturers to reformulate childhood vaccines in single-dose vials. It is interesting to note that even after children were immunized with thimerosal-free vaccines, a 2008 study from the California Department of Developmental Services showed that this action did not produce a decrease in autism rates [11]. Studies like this help to confirm the absence of an association between thimerosal and autism.

The two very large studies I reported on above for the MMR vaccine, namely, the Japanese case-control study and the meta-analysis, similarly found no link between vaccines containing thimerosal and autism [7, 8]. In addition, an earlier study published in *JAMA* in 2003 from the same Danish group that looked at the MMR vaccine also investigated vaccines that contained thimerosal [12]. During almost three million person years, they uncovered 440 autism cases and 787 cases of other autism spectrum disorders but found that the risk of both did not differ significantly between children immunized with vaccines containing thimerosal versus thimerosal-free vaccines. They also found that there was no evidence of a "dose-response association" between thimerosal and autism [12]. Similar to the California study, the Danish one further investigated autism rates following the discontinuation of Danish vaccines containing thimerosal, which had been used in childhood vaccines from the early 1950s up until 1992 [13]. They actually found that "discontinuation of thimerosal-containing vaccines in Denmark in 1992 was followed by an increase in the incidence of autism" [13]. It is likely that this finding does not reflect a true increased incidence but rather a reclassification of pediatric diagnoses from different disorders to ASD, but certainly discontinuation of thimerosal in no way led to a decrease in ASD, as would be expected if there was any causal association. My take on these studies is that even when pediatric vaccines contained thimerosal in the United States, they had no impact on the rates of autism or autism spectrum disorder.

In still another important study published in the *Proceedings of the National Academy of Sciences USA*, a group at the Infant Primate Research Laboratory in Seattle, together with a group based at the Department of Psychiatry of the University of Texas Southwestern Medical Center in Dallas, conducted an experimental study in which they injected infant rhesus macaques with vaccines that contained thimerosal, using the established vaccine schedules from either the 1990s or 2008 [14]. They examined the behavior of the macaques and conducted postmortem (autopsy) studies on their brains. The scientists found "no neuronal cellular or protein changes in the cerebellum, hippocampus, or amygdala" after administering vaccines that followed typical pediatric schedules. Also, there were "no significant differences in negative social behaviors between animals in the control and experimental groups." Their conclusion is that "[t]hese data indicate that administration of TCVs [thimerosal-containing vaccines] and/or MMR vaccine to rhesus macaques does not result in neuropathological abnormalities, or aberrant behaviors, like those observed in ASD" [14].

According to the CDC, currently the only major vaccine containing thimerosal routinely given to adults is the multi-dose influenza vaccine, which is also given to pregnant women [10]. Could this vaccine cause changes in the prenatal brain to produce autism [15]? I will have more to say about this in the next chapter.

The Upshot

An overwhelming body of evidence shows that pediatric vaccines routinely administered in childhood, including the MMR vaccine (implicated by the Wakefield group in the occurrence of autism) and thimerosal-containing vaccines, are not in any way linked with the disorder. They represent epidemiologic studies that were conducted in the most rigorous ways possible and that ultimately investigated more than one million vaccinated children. The studies were published in our leading, most prestigious, and most important rigorously peer-reviewed scientific journals, including the *New England Journal of Medicine, JAMA* and *JAMA Pediatrics, Proceedings of the National Academy of Sciences USA, Vaccine,* and the *Lancet.* They include retrospective cohort studies, case-control studies, meta-analysis studies, and experimental laboratory animal studies.

Most recently, some anti-vaccine groups have begun alleging links between the alum component of vaccines and autism. A 2018 PubMed search using the search terms "aluminum" and "autism" and "vaccine" over the last five years identifies eight articles purporting associations between alum-adjuvanted vaccines and autism. They include five written by a group at the University of British Columbia (UBC) and one at Keele University. The articles, which include reports on experimental studies in mice (including one which was subsequently retracted), are supported primarily by the Dwoskin Family Foundation and the Children's Medical Safety Research Institute as well as the Katlyn Fox Foundation, which has a mission of providing information "so that [parents] can make informed decisions on whether or not vaccines are suitable for their children" [16]. The Children's Medical Safety Research Institute was founded by Claire Dwoskin and (as of this writing) includes the UBC and Keele authors on their scientific advisory board. Alum is one of the oldest adjuvants found in vaccines and is currently used as an adjuvant in the DTaP, Hib, and hepatitis B vaccines, as well as in the newer pneumococcal conjugate vaccine. According to some estimates, alum has the world's "largest safety track record"—adjuvants have been given in more than three billion doses of vaccines over the past 80 years [17]. So far, there are no published retrospective-cohort or case-control epidemiological studies looking specifically at alum-containing vaccines and autism, similar to the MMR and thimerosal-containing vaccines (TVCs) studies highlighted above. Possibly this is because these latest alum assertions are still relatively new. However, the Australian meta-analysis showing that there is no association between autism and vaccines [8] included vaccines that contained alum. Moreover, as summarized above, there is no link between thimerosal-containing vaccines (TCVs) and autism [7], and the three major infant vaccines that previously comprised the TCVs—DTaP, hepatitis B, and Hib—are also formulated on alum. The Vaccine Education Center at Children's Hospital of Philadelphia further notes that "while infants receive 4.4 milligrams of aluminum in the first six months of life from vaccines, they receive more than that in their diet," with breast-fed infants ingesting approximately 7 mg, formula-fed infants 38 mg, and infants fed soy formula almost 117 mg [18].

As of 2018, when this book is scheduled to be published, I will have had my MD and PhD for more than 30 years. Over that time I have not seen anything close to this amount of scientific evidence refuting a causal association between an intervention and a medical condition. In my opinion, efforts to study autism and its possible relationship with vaccines rank among the most thorough investigations in all of biomedical science. From my perspective, there is no ambiguity. The science clearly finds there is no association between vaccines and ASD. Today, the anti-vaccine groups still attempt to refute these findings. They do so in interesting ways such as trying find mistakes in the methodologies or even resorting to conspiracy theories stating that the papers are fake news. By persisting in these actions, they are doing a disservice to children and adults with autism and their families.

· 9 ·

What Does Cause Autism?

THE SCIENTIFIC EVIDENCE

As detailed in the previous chapter, a massive amount of evidence refutes any links between vaccines and autism. We now have data and information on more than one million children that show vaccines do *not* cause autism, including the MMR vaccine given to children, vaccines that previously contained thimerosal, or any other vaccine studied to date. But there is another important part to this story. As the father of a child with autism, I would also like to point out that there is no reasonable *plausibility* of vaccines causing autism. I can assert this with confidence because we now know so much more about the genetic and neurobiological complexities of autism than ever before. All of this new information reinforces the lack of any association between vaccines and autism and indeed points toward the realization that any vaccine given during childhood simply could not cause it. The brains of kids with autism are so different in terms of their anatomy and structure, both at the visible and the microscopic levels, that there is no reasonable way we could account for those effects as being caused by a vaccine given in infancy or early childhood. Instead, the brains of kids (and of course, ultimately, adults) with autism are structurally different from those of people without autism, and these changes almost certainly begin prenatally—before the child is born.

A Second Wave of Scientific Evidence

Autism, of course, comprises a wide range of conditions, and that's why it is often referred to as autism spectrum disorder (ASD). It's difficult to account for all of the variations. Today, ASD incorporates a number of conditions that previously went by different names, including PDD-NOS, Asperger's syndrome, and autistic disorder [1]. In our case, Rachel was diagnosed as having developmental delays at 18–20 months of age, which were ultimately shown to be linked with ASD. This is the typical time when children are diagnosed with ASD. The CDC website describes the following scenario: "Some children with an ASD seem to develop normally until around 18 to 24 months of age and then they stop gaining new skills, or they lose the skills they once had. Studies have shown that one-third to half of parents of children with an ASD noticed a problem before their child's first birthday, and nearly 80%–90% saw problems by 24 months of age" [1].

So, most parents commonly observe behaviors linked to ASD when their children are somewhere between one and two years of age. As the CDC points out, such behaviors can manifest by either an arrest in development when they either stop gaining skills or gain them at a lower rate, or a regressive form of autism in which they actually lose skills and fall behind milestones in child development. A paper from the MIND Institute at the University of California, Davis—an important Sacramento-based institute devoted to ASD and other neurodevelopmental disorders—termed this "regressive autism." Regressive autism, which also occurs during the second year of life, is associated with loss of communication and social skills [2]. Two of Rachel's child psychiatrists—Dr. Fred Volkmar and the late Dr. Donald Cohen—are credited as being among the first to recognize this form of ASD [3], along with groups from Japan [4].

The Neurobiology of ASD

The Global Burden of Disease Study (GBD) 2015, which I previously mentioned for its role in measuring the dramatic declines in child mortality from vaccine-preventable diseases as a result of the Millennial Development Goals and Gavi, the Vaccine Alliance, also estimates that 62.2 million people live with ASD, including 24.8 million classified as having "autism" and 37.2 million with "Asperger syndrome and other autistic spectrum disorders." [5]. As the classifications change, we can expect further revisions of these estimates in the coming years. Another estimate from the GBD is that autism is associated with 10 million years lived with disability (YLDs). YLDs are useful, because they allow one to compare the global level of disability of different conditions. To put such numbers in perspective, the 10 million YLDs from autism are about one-third those resulting from diabetes (33.4 million YLDs) and significantly greater than the disability level from Alzheimer's disease and other dementias (6.8 million YLDs) [5]. The bottom line is that the GBD confirms a devastating disease burden resulting from ASD.

How were autism and ASD discovered? A PubMed search of the biomedical literature using the term "autism" reveals that the first scientific article to use it came from Dr. Leo Kanner in a 1946 paper published in the *American Journal of Psychiatry* titled "Irrelevant and Metaphorical Language in Early

Infantile Autism." [6] However, it's possible to find reference to an earlier publication by Kanner from 1943 titled "Autistic Disturbances to Affective Contact." Kanner is also an important historical figure in American psychiatry. He was an Austrian-born Jewish psychiatrist who fled Weimar Germany during the 1920s (before Hitler came to power). During the 1930s, he helped to launch one of the first child psychiatry programs in the United States, based at Johns Hopkins University and hospital.

An early observation made by first Kanner, then reported in detail during the 1990s [7–9] and subsequently confirmed by groups at the University of California at San Diego (UCSD) and Los Angeles (UCLA) [10, 11], is that children with ASD often have large heads—a condition referred to as macrocephaly. Moreover, the enlarged heads of kids with autism are associated with the overgrowth of parts of the brain [10, 11]. In a paper published in *JAMA* in 2003, the UCSD group, headed by Dr. Eric Courchesne, noted the increase in head size occurs in two major waves during the first two years of life. An area that is particularly affected was found to be the cerebral cortex, the outer neural layer of the major part of the brain that controls our thoughts and language, among other critical higher functions [11]. Such studies highlighted that there are important anatomic or structural changes to the brains of children with ASD.

In early 2017, an important follow-up paper appeared in the prestigious journal *Nature* that helps to explain both the expanding head size and brain overgrowth and why the full clinical expression of ASD seems to occur in the 18- to 24-month-old time frame highlighted by the CDC [12–14]. A group led by Dr. Joe Piven at the University of North Carolina–Chapel Hill conducted imaging studies of the brain through magnetic resonance imaging (MRI) and noted that brain volume over-growth occurs between 12 and 24 months in children diag-nosed with ASD at 24 months. In other words, brain volume overgrowth coincides with or shortly precedes the clinical ex-pression of autism. The Piven group reported that brain vol-ume overgrowth "was linked to the emergence and severity of autistic social deficits" [13].

This finding is very important because it is at around this time that so many parents (including Ann and me) recognize autistic behaviors in their children and first seek medical at-tention. The period between one and two years of age is when brain volume increases and ASD is frequently diagnosed. That same period is also an important time in a child's routine vac-cine schedule. According to the CDC, in the United States and elsewhere, children are expected to receive during this period at least one of the doses in the series of their routine childhood vaccines, including their MMR and varicella vaccines; a dose of the diphtheria, tetanus, and acellular pertussis vaccine; rota-virus vaccine; and often their inactivated polio vaccine [15].

Given that this period temporally coincides with the age at which children are commonly diagnosed with autism (includ-ing the regressive form), it is not surprising to me that some parents might link the two events together. The fact that chil-dren often cry when they receive vaccines reinforces this sup-position. In our case, Rachel would cry longer and with much fiercer intensity than our other children. When children on the autism spectrum receive their vaccines, this can become both an unpleasant and very memorable event.

So is it possible that the vaccines given between one and two years of age are triggering the brain volume overgrowth leading to the clinical signs of ASD? The answer is a pretty emphatic no, at least according to the *Nature* paper. Instead, the UNC–Chapel Hill team found that the MRI data showed that the period of brain volume overgrowth in the one- to two-year-olds is actually preceded by a 6- to 12-month period of hyperexpansion of the cortical surface of the brain [13]. In other words, the changes in the brains of kids with ASD are set into motion well before (about a year) many parents recognize any signs of alterations in communication or social behavior. The authors conclude: "The rate of cortical surface area expansion from 6 to 12 months was significantly increased in individuals diagnosed with autism at 24 months, and was linked to subsequent brain overgrowth, which, in turn, was linked to the emergence of social deficits. This suggests a sequence whereby hyperexpansion of the cortical surface area is an early event in a cascade leading to brain overgrowth and emerging autistic deficits" [13].

In a subsequent paper published in the prestigious journal *Science Translational Medicine*, the Piven group was able to use this information to predict with more than 90 percent accuracy whether a 6-month-old infant will develop autism at 24 months of age. Specifically, they reported: "Functional brain connections were defined in 6-month-old infants that correlated with 24-month scores on measures of social behavior, language, motor development, and repetitive behavior, which are all features common to the diagnosis of ASD" [14]. Such information runs counter to the assertion by some parents that autism or ASD begins after receiving vaccines in the second year of life. While they might have recognized that their children were autistic or even began regressing in behavior between one and two years of age, especially between 18 and 24 months, the science shows that their autism destiny was already set in motion at least one year previously. The researchers emphasize that "[t]hese findings must be replicated, but they represent an important step toward the early identification of individuals with autism before its characteristic symptoms develop" [14]. In other words, it should now be possible to predict by 6 months of age whether or not a child will exhibit signs of ASD by 24 months of age.

Prenatal Development

Recently, additional evidence suggests that the changes in the brains of children with ASD begin even earlier than at 6–12 months old and actually start before birth—during prenatal development. In 2014, Courchesne's UCSD group published an important paper in the *New England Journal of Medicine* based on postmortem (autopsy) studies of children with ASD. Specifically, they identified patches of disorganized cerebral cortex in the prefrontal cortex and temporal lobes, which are regions of the brain responsible for communication, language, and social functions—all known to be disrupted in ASD (fig. 7). However, the processes leading to the disorganization of these areas of the brain are believed to have been set in motion before birth. They write, "Such abnormalities may represent a common set of developmental neuropathological features that underlie autism and probably result from dysregulation of layer formation and layer-specific neuronal differentiation at prenatal developmental stages" [16].

A major point is that in children with ASD there are changes in the brain of the developing fetus, well before a child receives his or her first vaccination. These changes in the brain tissue begin before birth and subsequently lead to cortical surface expansion at 6 to 12 months, and then brain volume overgrowth at 12 to 24 months, when the clinical expression of autism is most evident. Possibly, we can now predict by 6 months of age

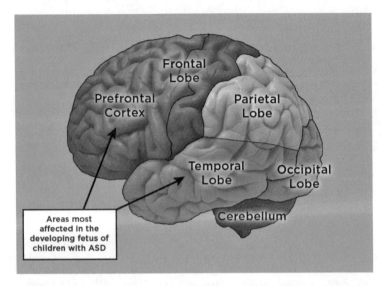

FIGURE 7. Areas of the brain most affected in children with autism spectrum disorder.

Source: Hotez PJ (2017). Autism spectrum disorder: If not vaccines, then what? Baylor College of Medicine, From the Labs (blog), February 24. https://from thelabs.bcm.edu/2017/02/24/autism-spectrum-disorder-if-not-vaccinesthen-what.

whether a child will develop ASD, but the Courchesne findings suggest we might soon be able to predict autism at birth or even prenatally.

Genetics

So what first triggers the alterations of the cortical layers in the prefrontal and temporal regions of the brain as described by Courchesne's group? There is a lot of evidence pointing to altered genes—changes to the DNA either through point mutations or even deletions of entire regions of DNA.

A recent paper published in *Nature Neuroscience* by groups from the Simons Foundation and Princeton University describes some of these genetic changes [17]. Unfortunately, the genetics of ASD is not a straightforward story—or, as the authors point out, autism genetics is highly complex and even "daunting." Ultimately, the authors believe, up to 1,000 different genes might one day be identified as being responsible for ASD, and so far only 65 of those genes have been found [17]. Such findings help explain the greatly increased risk of ASD among children born in families in which a biologic sibling was diagnosed with autism [18, 19].

The Princeton University–Simons Foundation group has now incorporated the 65 known ASD genes and used modern computational biology methods to build one of the first networks of interacting genes. Most of them are linked to changes in the cerebral cortex happening at the early or mid-fetal stage of development [17]. This means that genes are directly causing the prenatal changes in the brain previously described by Courchesne and his colleagues. These researchers report, "Our analysis identified a clear developmental pattern—a prenatal signal from the early, mid and late fetal stages—indicating that autism associated genetic changes affect the development of the fetal prefrontal, temporal and cerebellar cortex" [17].

These findings point strongly to a genetic basis of ASD and events that begin in prenatal development. They also potentially point to the promise of designing specific interventions and small molecule drugs that could one day counteract some of the deleterious genes or gene products that cause ASD in its severest form. Some of these efforts are being led by my colleague Dr. Huda Zoghbi, who heads the Neurological Research Institute based at Texas Children's Hospital and Baylor College of Medicine and has done pioneering work on the regressive form of autism associated with Rett syndrome [20]. Clearly, if we want to make an impact on ASD, unravel all 1,000 genes, and begin to think about a cure, we need to invest heavily in the science of autism genetics.

In 2017, Ann and I arranged with the Department of Genetics at Baylor College of Medicine to sequence our DNA as well as Rachel's DNA. Whole exome sequencing (WES) is a process in which the full sequences of all of the genes that encode proteins are obtained. The goal of WES is to identify any genetic mutations or deletions in our genes that might alter protein sequences—in this case, any of the known genes or proteins that so far have been linked to ASD or intellectual disabilities. This information could be useful for identifying unique proteins that could be targeted for medication or treatment, but also it could inform Rachel's siblings about their risks for having children with mental disabilities. Unfortunately, the yield for identifying alterations in autism genes is not high, because there may be almost 1,000 genes for autism and we have only identified about 65 of them.

Ann and I were a little apprehensive about the conducting of WES. What if it revealed something unexpected or terrible about us, or our family, or about Rachel? Also we were concerned about collateral damage—WES might inform us that we're at greater risk of Alzheimer's disease or other end-of-life conditions. Indeed, it turns out that Rachel had some genetic variants, including one affecting a gene that could be linked to ASD or mental disabilities. To try and pin this association down we're planning to add Rachel's new genetic information to an initiative run jointly between Baylor and Johns Hopkins—The Baylor Johns Hopkins Center for Mendelian

Genetics—in order to determine if Rachel's genetic variants might also be present in other individuals on the autism spectrum or with other mental health conditions. In addition, we plan to link Rachel's new findings to the Undiagnosed Diseases Network, a large US National Institutes of Health–supported study that brings together institutions across the country and is coordinated at Harvard Medical School. We still have a long way to go, but we feel there's real hope that a genetic basis for Rachel's autism might be identified, and maybe even a possibility that these findings could reveal potential targets for therapeutic intervention.

Epigenetics and Prenatal Environmental Effects

While genes and genetic factors influencing the neurodevelopment of the cortical layers of the cerebral cortex, especially the prefrontal and temporal lobes, probably represent the major mechanism(s) by which ASD occurs, there are potential additional factors at play. An important influence is the role of epigenetics, a rapidly growing field of modern science, which refers to how genes are modified, especially in very early pregnancy, at or around the time of conception. While not nearly as familiar to the general public as genetics, epigenetics is an exciting and recent area of molecular biology and genetics and is based on findings that go beyond alterations in the actual genetic material—DNA—of an individual through mutations in the DNA or DNA deletions. Instead, epigenetics deals with how genes, altered or otherwise, are regulated or expressed in order to influence an individual's characteristics, possibly including areas relevant to autism such as social interactions, communications, and language. To date, several important molecular mechanisms underlying epigenetics have been identified, including methylation of DNA, modifications in the regulatory proteins that interact with DNA such as histones or repressors, and an important and still little-understood role for unusual RNA molecules known as non-coding RNAs or micro RNAs (mRNAs) that may turn on, silence, or otherwise regulate genes [12]. Epigenetics is likely to also have an important role in the events leading to ASD and autism. Again, we need significant investments in the science of autism epigenetics.

Possibly through epigenetic or as still yet undefined mechanisms, certain prenatal exposures or environmental factors, such as specific chemical toxins in the environment or even congenital infectious agents, may cause abnormal fetal development leading to ASD. In 2010, Dr. Phil Landrigan, a distinguished environmental health expert and epidemiologist from the Mount Sinai School of Medicine in New York, wrote a comprehensive overview paper that summarized the known exposures that could cause multiple fetal abnormalities that include the altered behaviors associated with higher social functions, communications, and language that constitute ASD [21].

A particularly interesting exposure cited by Landrigan is the rubella virus, which can cause a congenital rubella syndrome (CRS), characterized by ocular cataracts, deafness, and heart defects, as well as neurodevelopmental delays that can closely resemble autism. CRS has largely disappeared in the United States through widespread vaccination; as a medical student in New York, I remember seeing only one case of CRS. The irony here is that the "R" component of the MMR vaccine is actually the rubella vaccine that protects a mother from transmitting rubella virus to her baby, and in so doing functions as an effective vaccine *against* autism. Recently, Dr. Ian Lipkin and his colleagues at Columbia University have also found that maternal herpes simplex virus type 2 (HSV-2) may also be linked to autism [22], although from my perspective, the association does not appear to be as strong as the rubella link. However, the Lipkin group has found that maternal fever, especially multiple fevers or fever in the second trimester of pregnancy could be linked to ASD. Such findings provide further support for maternal infections during early pregnancy in promoting autism [23].

The Landrigan paper further identifies chemical toxins in the environment that could also lead to ASD or ASD-like behaviors, especially when they are associated with prolonged or heavy exposures during early pregnancy [21]. They include drugs or chemicals such as valproic acid, a neuropsychiatric medicine that helps with mood stabilization, an organophosphate insecticide known as chlorpyrifos, thalidomide, and misoprostol, among others. In contrast, the Landrigan paper rules out vaccines. But what about vaccines given to pregnant women—could they be somehow linked to autism? The short answer, in my view, is an emphatic no, but the details are worth a discussion.

Emory University's Dr. Saad Omer has recently reviewed the major vaccines given during pregnancy, most notably maternal influenza vaccination and pertussis vaccination in the form of Tdap. Other maternal vaccines are also under development and could one day include vaccines for respiratory syncytial virus (RSV) and group B streptococcus [24]. Of the two major maternal immunizations currently in use, Tdap is typically administered late in pregnancy, and because the brains of children with ASD are already well developed by that point, I don't see a likelihood that this vaccine plays a role in the disorder. In contrast, influenza vaccine could be given at any point during a pregnancy, including the first trimester.

In 2017, a research group at Kaiser Permanente Northern California in Oakland conducted a decade-long study of almost 200,000 children born into its health plan to look at the effects of maternal flu immunization. Their overall finding was that "[t]here was no association between maternal influenza infection anytime during pregnancy and increased ASD risk." However, they did find a 1.2 odds ratio indicating "there was a suggestion of increased ASD risk among children whose mothers received an influenza vaccination in their first trimester, but the association was not statistically significant after adjusting for multiple comparisons, indicating that the finding could be due to chance" [25]. To put this number in further perspective, it turns out that some of the studies highlighted in the previous chapter showing no associations between childhood immunizations and autism, actually exhibit odds ratios in the 0.8 to 0.9 range. Such numbers indicate that at some level vaccines may actually protect somewhat against autism. But because these numbers are not statistically significant, we cannot make such claims.

You might ask, if the finding of maternal flu vaccine and autism was not statistically significant why raise it at all? I do so because maternal flu vaccine is in some cases still administered from multi-dose vials that contain thimerosal. And in response to the Kaiser Permanente study, Dr. Janet Kern submitted a comment to *JAMA Pediatrics* making the point that there were flaws in the statistical methods used in the study [26]. But from my viewpoint, if there really was an important association, we would not be seeing such a modest and statistically insignificant increase, such as an odds ratio of 1.2. Instead, for a real association we would be looking at numbers far higher, and certainly exceeding 2 or 3, if not more. For me, it is clear there is no association, but moving forward I think it's possible we will eventually begin to immunize potentially pregnant women only with single-dose influenza vaccines that do not contain thimerosal. More important, we need to explore in more detail the few actual environmental toxins—chemicals and infectious agents—that have been linked to ASD, including those highlighted by Landrigan and his colleagues. Such an effort would include identifying mechanisms by which these chemicals and infections interact with the 65 or more ASD genes so far identified.

I'm very much baffled by groups that keep revisiting thimerosal-autism links rather than focusing on the half-dozen chemicals that when used in pregnancy clearly do have an association. I find it terribly frustrating that we have massive data showing the genetic or epigenetic basis of autism, together with a handful of environmental toxins, and yet the anti-vaccine groups continue to perseverate on factors that have no association or any plausibility. From my standpoint, the anti-vaccine movement ranks among the most self-defeating anti-science movements in America or globally.

The Upshot

Figure 8 summarizes the events leading to ASD, which I highlighted above. Briefly, like Rachel, children with ASD frequently are diagnosed with developmental delays or regression between one and two years of age, but especially between 18 and 24 months. This period coincides with a significant amount of brain volume overgrowth and macrocephaly and can be linked to either a stoppage of developmental milestones or, less commonly, can manifest as a regression of social, communication, and language skills. While some parents note that period can roughly coincide with a time when their child

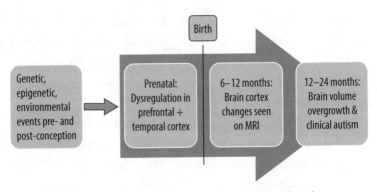

FIGURE 8. Sequence of events leading to autism spectrum disorder.

Source: Hotez PJ (2017). Autism spectrum disorder: If not vaccines, then what? Baylor College of Medicine, From the Labs (blog), February 24. https://from thelabs.bcm.edu/2017/02/24/autism-spectrum-disorder-if-not-vaccines-then -what.

received vaccinations, the UNC–Chapel Hill group has shown that changes in the MRIs of these children actually began a year before. Equally important is the finding by the UCSD group that even these changes are preceded by alterations or dysregulation of the cortical layer in the prefrontal and temporal lobes of the brains of children with ASD during early pregnancy. ASD begins prenatally—during pregnancy.

Finally, such prenatal events seem to be triggered by genetic alternations—mutations or deletions—in at least 65 genes, possibly together with epigenetic events linked to alterations in gene expression. In some cases there may be chemical toxins or infectious diseases in the environment that interact with these genes or epigenetic factors and contribute to these early prenatal events. But the bottom line is that none of the sequence of events leading to ASD relies on vaccines or vaccinations.

· 10 ·

Struck by Lightning

As the overwhelming evidence now shows that vaccines do not cause autism, I've observed the anti-vaccine community begin attempting to link vaccines to other illnesses, disease conditions, or symptoms. These include various neuropsychological disturbances that were recently surveyed by a group of experts based at the CDC, together with other university-based investigators, who examined abnormalities in the following areas: "[g]eneral intellectual function, speech and language, verbal memory, attention and executive function, tics, achievement, visual spatial ability, and behavior regulation" [1, 2]. Two studies were conducted. First, based on concerns raised by some parent groups that children are exposed to too many vaccines, the CDC analyzed the effects of thousands of antigen doses administered among a large group of children who had received immunizations during the first two years of life and were then studied 7 to 10 years later. The CDC findings are quite clear: "We did not find any adverse associations between antigens received through vaccines in the first two years of life and neuropsychological outcomes in later childhood" [1].

In a second study focusing on the role of thimerosal-containing vaccines (as well as immune globulins), some of the same authors conducted a neuropsychological assessment at 7 to 10 years of children who had received these immunizations early in life. They looked at the same parameters as the other study, including "intellectual functioning, speech and language, verbal memory, executive functioning, fine motor coordination, tics and behavior regulation." They found no impact of thimerosal on six of the seven neuropsychological outcomes. However, they noted a "small, but statistically significant association between early thimerosal exposure and the presence of tics in boys," but not in girls [2].

Other studies have also looked at the possible relationship between exposure to thimerosal-containing vaccines and tics, with some showing an association, others not. Given that the overall frequency of tics is very low, the variation in results is not too surprising. Such associations often suggest that they might occur through chance alone. As a pediatric infectious diseases physician, I have seen a similar question arise when it comes to determining whether a particular microbial pathogen is linked to a specific disease syndrome. For instance, the microorganism known as *Blastocystis hominis* has been shown in some studies to be linked to diarrheal disease and other gastrointestinal disturbances, while others refute an association [3]. Specifically regarding tics, the CDC authors' major finding was that a potential association between vaccines and tics in boys should "be interpreted with caution due to limitations in the measurement of tics and the limited biological plausibility regarding a causal relationship" [2]. I think this relationship deserves further study, maybe with larger numbers of children and perhaps with better case definitions for tics. But overall, I'm skeptical that a link between tics and vaccines will hold up.

I'm similarly skeptical about a case-controlled study published in 2017 by doctors and scientists from Wisconsin's

Marshfield Clinic, the CDC, and Kaiser Permanente showing that during the years 2010–11 and 2011–12, spontaneous abortion (miscarriage) was associated with maternal influenza vaccination (containing a 2009 H1N1 antigen) within the preceding 28 days [4]. It's interesting to note that the authors do not believe there is a causal link, given that many other studies have not demonstrated the connection and there are other potential explanations [4]. For example, some have suggested that high-risk pregnancy patients are more likely to be vaccinated, among several other reasons [5]. Alternatively, Dr. Paul Offit points out the small number of cases in the study and notes that the risk of spontaneous abortion was found only in those who were vaccinated two years in a row; if they hadn't been vaccinated in the previous year, there was no added risk [6]. Indeed a follow-up study conducted by some of the same authors confirmed there was no link during 2009–10, when pregnant women were vaccinated with both seasonal and pandemic H1N1 flu strains [7].

Whack-a-Mole

My hope is that this book can help to slow national and international anti-vaccine movements, especially the prominent wings that allege vaccines cause autism. My premise is that the American anti-vaccine movement has grown and become well organized based on a toxic combination of hysteria and pseudoscience. However, I'm also starting to see that public engagement with the anti-vaccine movement is a bit like the arcade game of whack-a-mole, in which knocking down the different claims that vaccines cause autism results in a new or alternative allegation. For example, knocking down the assertion that MMR vaccines cause autism stimulated allegations about thimerosal; closing that avenue stimulated an assertion that vaccines are administered too closely together in time.

Of late, we're now starting to see yet a new crop of alleged negative or unhealthy things that vaccines do to kids. They include assertions of other neurodevelopmental defects that go beyond autism, which were debunked in the discussion above. But that may be just the beginning. Some parents groups now allege vaccines cause food allergies, autoimmune disorders, multiple sclerosis, and a number of other adverse health conditions.

In June 2017, and in a strange twist, the Court of Justice of the European Union ruled that the courts may link vaccines to illnesses even if the findings are not supported by scientific evidence. The ruling was based on the case of a man from France who received his hepatitis B vaccine in 1998, developed multiple sclerosis the following year, and died in 2011 [8]. To date, there is no proven link or even any plausible connection between hepatitis B vaccine and multiple sclerosis, but still the courts can presumably concoct causes and effects that fly in the face of science. Similar faux links have been alleged in the context of the new cervical cancer vaccine for human papillomavirus. However, according to Paul Offit and others there is no epidemiological evidence to support such contentions [9, 10].

The Vaccine Adverse Events Reporting System

In order to gather as much information as possible about potential side effects or vaccine toxicities, in 1990 the US CDC and FDA established an effective and timely Vaccine Adverse Events Reporting System (VAERS) as a "national early warning system" to monitor potential or actual side effects for licensed vaccines in the United States. The major objectives of VAERS are to "detect new, unusual, or rare vaccine adverse events," monitor any increases in these events, determine risk factors linked to adverse events, and evaluate the overall safety of new vaccines [11]. VAERS is positioned so that it can also identify specific lots of vaccine that may be defective, contaminated, or responsible for unusual side effects or adverse events [11].

Adverse events reporting and monitoring is especially important for newly licensed vaccines and ones just being introduced into the US population. For example, when the US vaccine manufacturer Wyeth Laboratories introduced a new rotavirus vaccine (Rotashield) in the summer of 1999, VAERS picked up a rare gastrointestinal complication known as intussusception, a condition in which one part of the intestine collapses into another to cause potential gastrointestinal obstruction [12]. Intussusception was found in 15 infants who had received their first vaccine dose [11, 12]. In response and in consultation with the FDA, Wyeth voluntarily withdrew the vaccine and halted its distribution, while ACIP reviewed the data. Ultimately, ACIP confirmed the link between Rotashield and intussusception and then withdrew its recommendation for the vaccine [12]. From my standpoint, these events provide proof-of-concept that monitoring by VAERS is robust and can pick up important vaccine side effects if and when they occur.

Over the 10-year period between 2006 and 2015, almost three billion doses of vaccine have been provided in the United States—or roughly 300 million doses annually [13]. Of those 300 million doses of vaccines, VAERS estimates that it receives about 30,000 reports annually, equivalent to 0.01 percent of vaccinations [14]. Approximately one-third of these reports come from health-care providers, while an equal number come from the vaccine manufacturers themselves [11]. The rest are received from parents or guardians, state immunization programs, and other sources [15].

Of these 30,000 reports to VAERS, approximately 85–90 percent are considered mild adverse events, described as "fever, arm soreness, and crying or mild irritability" [14]. In contrast, roughly 15 percent (about 3,000–4,500 vaccination reports annually) involve "hospitalization, permanent disability, or death, which may or may not have been caused by a vaccine" [16]. That last phrase is an important part of the statement, because these serious adverse events are followed up by the CDC and FDA to determine if they were actually linked to the vaccine. According to VAERS, the system "accepts reports of adverse events following vaccination without judging the cause or seriousness of the event. Some adverse events might be caused by vaccination and others might be coincidental and not related to vaccination. Just because an adverse event happened after a person received a vaccine does not mean the vaccine caused the adverse event. VAERS is not designed to determine if a vaccine caused an adverse event, but it is good at detecting unusual or unexpected patterns of reporting that might indicate possible safety problems that need a closer look" [15].

The major serious but rare adverse events linked to vaccines currently include anaphylaxis (severe allergic reaction), shoulder or local neurologic injury at the injection site, seizures from fever that can result from a vaccination (febrile seizure), and fainting [17, 18]. Very rarely, encephalopathy, encephalitis, or other life-threatening syndromes or illnesses can result, which can occur especially if a live virus vaccine is administered by mistake to an individual with severe immune deficiency. Such an individual should be medically exempted from receiving live virus vaccines.

So exactly how many of the 3,000-odd serious adverse events out of 300 million vaccine doses (1 in 100,000, or 0.001 percent) are actually caused by vaccines? According to VAERS, "While these problems happen after vaccination, they are rarely caused by the vaccine" [14]. To try to get our arms around a more specific number, we can also look to a second system of checks and balances put into place by the US government.

The National Vaccine Injury Compensation Program

There are extremely rare instances when vaccines can cause a severe allergic reaction or other severe adverse events. To provide fair financial compensation for such injuries, NVICP was created during the 1980s to provide an alternative to lawsuits against vaccine manufacturers and pediatricians and other health-care providers who administer vaccines [19]. A major rationale was that the threat of lawsuits was beginning to drive the major multinational pharmaceutical companies that make vaccines out of that business. This is because the major vaccine companies, such as GlaxoSmithKline, Merck, Sanofi-Pasteur, and Pfizer, actually receive only a modest percentage of their profits and return on investment from vaccine sales (compared, say, with drugs for lowering cholesterol or blood pressure that have to be taken daily), so withdrawing from vaccine markets might not have a substantial impact on their shareholders. At one point there was a real possibility that we could lose most of our global vaccine manufacturing capacity.

Currently, any individual (or his or her guardian) who receives a vaccine recommended by the CDC/ACIP and feels that the vaccine resulted in injury can file a petition with NVIC [19]. Over a 20-year period between 1988 and 2017, approximately 18,000 vaccine-related claims were filed, of which 11,000 were dismissed and almost 5,500 received some sort of compensation [13].

To put those numbers in perspective, over a 20-year period, almost 300 serious adverse events annually were linked by NVICP in some way to actually receiving a vaccine. It can be argued that in actuality there were more than 300 adverse events for which petitions were not filed or that were unfairly adjudicated, but it can be equally argued that not all of those 300 adverse events were definitively linked to vaccines. But using that 300 number and the 300 million doses of vaccines given annually (estimated above), the likelihood of severe injury from vaccines is roughly 1 in 1,000,000. To put that number in perspective, some estimate that the odds of being struck by lightning in any one year are 1 in 700,000 [20].

In order to qualify for receiving compensation from NVICP, one of three criteria needs to be met, including injury lasting at least six months, injury resulting in hospitalization or requiring surgery, or injury resulting in death [21]. There must be proof that such injuries are related to a CDC/ACIP-approved vaccine. NVICP has also received claims for autism resulting from either MMR or thimerosal-containing vaccine. Such claims began in 2001, and in 2002 a special Omnibus Autism Program was created. Over the course of the next decade, 5,600 claims were filed, with 4,800 pending and 800 claims dismissed [21]. It is possible that some or many of the dismissed cases are now going through the conventional tort system.

If NVICP were to routinely award injury compensation due to ASD, one can only imagine its potential total cost. According to the CDC, approximately 1 in 68 children is on the autism spectrum [22]. My back-of-the-envelope calculation says that if approximately 75 million children live in the United States, we're looking at more than one million children with ASD, so that opening the door to compensation for children with ASD could easily reach the trillion dollar level and bankrupt NVICP. In other words, payout for ASD could one day exceed the Tobacco Master Settlement Agreement with the four large US tobacco companies.

Some of my colleagues allege that the potential for such payouts has incentivized plaintive attorneys (or groups linked to them) to help finance anti-vaccine lobbies, groups, or even prominent individuals. They contend that such financial support has sustained anti-vaccine groups for the past two decades. While I suppose this is possible, I have no firsthand evidence for it. But the idea might be worthy of future investigation.

· 11 ·

Our Family's Future

Rachel is no longer in the Houston school system, and she seems to lack the level of compliance and cooperation that is required for gainful employment. It's been a huge challenge to find her a job. Rachel is now going on 25 years of age, and even young adults with far fewer verbal skills are likely to be more successful in terms of holding down any type of employment. Even though there is no question that Rachel has her charms, unless there is a big change, it's difficult for us to imagine how an employer would put up with her attention deficits, rigidity, and oppositional attitudes, especially on top of her intellectual disabilities. At least in the beginning, Rachel will require a lot of intensive support.

While I'm at the Texas Medical Center during the day, Ann makes heroic efforts to vary Rachel's routine and fold in some meaningful stimulation. There are the trips to the dentist and doctor, but Ann also tries to structure visits with age-appropriate adults. Ann is an amazing advocate for Rachel and tries all sorts of special needs programs offered across the city of Houston, but most of them don't seem to work out for one reason or another. In the programs for high-functioning young adults or those able to maintain employment, Rachel lacks the compliance and drive to make it work. In the programs for severely impaired young adults, Rachel gets frustrated and doesn't receive the social stimulation she craves. As a result, so far she has fallen through the cracks. As of this writing, Rachel has just begun job training at Goodwill. We're cautiously excited about this possibility. Goodwill is providing a job coach, which will be funded by Social Security insurance through the Texas Department of Assistive and Rehabilitative Services (DARS) to help her stay on task, while she sorts donated clothes. We're holding our breaths and crossing our fingers, because Ann and I are pretty desperate for Rachel to find some type of job placement in our neighborhood.

Many parts of our life are better in Texas. I have a dream job, our finances are under control, and we're out of financial debt for the first time. Dan, our youngest son, moved with us to Houston and is now studying to become a petroleum engineer at the University of Oklahoma. I'm somewhat apprehensive about what happened to our city during Hurricane Harvey and how it will recover over time, but generally I'm quite upbeat about our life here. Houstonians are pretty resilient. Even though both Ann and I live far from our extended families in the Northeast, they are also making a good effort to stay connected to Rachel. These days, Rachel phones Julie and other family members on a daily basis.

But we worry about Rachel's future. We're anxious to find a meaningful life for her. We're also realistic. Even if she finally lands a job through DARS and Goodwill, we know that many of their clients cannot maintain their employment. The reasons for this are myriad and include problems like getting to work on time, following rules, or maintaining a strict schedule. Even the most basic jobs require many skills and self-discipline, which normally developing people may hardly recognize as such. Ultimately, a sizable number wind up living at home and unemployed.

Ann and I are getting older, and we see a time when we won't be around anymore. Will Rachel remain employed? Can she ever live on her own? If not, then what? Worry and anxiety about Rachel's future is always with us and is a source of constant tension in our lives. Overall, the safety net for adults on the autism spectrum is not strong in our state—nor is it nationally. I wish the debate surrounding autism would focus less on vaccines and more on real and everyday urgencies.

Ann describes our situation and sentiments with sensitivity and brave honesty:

> I think every parent of a special needs child worries about who will care for their adult child when they are not here anymore. Peter and I have no answers, but we are starting to think more systematically about this heart-wrenching planning for our adult child. ARC, the national organization for people with disabilities, has an online toolkit to help parents organize, and I am just about ready to tackle that.
>
> My father used to say that the six questions to ask in journalism were who, what, when, where, why—and perhaps most important, how?
>
> Unfortunately, Peter and I are nowhere near answering any of those questions. We look around and see that some families have built homes for their adult children housed within specialized communities. Others have created businesses for their kids to run. We're now addressing legalities such as special needs trust and guardianship legalities, which encompass other members of the family, including siblings. It is daunting, to say the least, and Peter and I need to step

up and get some control over this scary future. For now, we have a sometimes disheveled, beautiful red-haired girl who is full of questions and ideas about what she would like to eat at her next meal, when she will next see her friend Sabrina, where she will celebrate her birthday, and when she will visit her Aunt Julie in Washington, DC.

Those questions we can answer; however, so many others we cannot.

More recently, we have had a glimmer of hope and optimism. While waiting to board an airplane in the fall of 2017, Peter and I met a smart and engaging woman, and our initially lighthearted conversation rather quickly turned to Rachel. We mentioned that our daughter was not having any success at finding any type of job, and we were very surprised to learn that we were speaking to Melinda Kacal of the Portland, Oregon, Goodwill foundation, married to Bill Kacal, senior chairman of the board at Goodwill Houston. Major changes were in store for Rachel, as Melinda quickly conveyed to Bill the disheartening situation we were facing. They helped us to overcome the previous barrier that Rachel has had to any employment, which was attaining a job coach to work beside her and guide her—someone to help her learn to do the job and to stay on task. Bill and Melinda arranged a meeting with us to meet Alma Ybarra, the director of workforce development, and Steve Luftburrow, president and CEO of Goodwill Houston.

From that meeting, Rachel was promptly enrolled in Goodwill training classes for four consecutive Mondays and job coaching for two hours a day. Reyna Garces, a job skills trainer, compassionately but firmly guides Rachel, training her as a sorter. More specifically, she is instructed to find rips and stains in clothing and she is taught to work slowly so that she does not miss those stains! She receives a paycheck electronically, which is puzzling to her but very exciting. Rachel is truly beyond thrilled! She is finally earning some of her own money and is always asking us how much she has earned so far! I tell her, working two hours a day and after taxes, it is about $14 a day and $215 so far. Peter and I are just pinching ourselves over our good luck, how our chance meeting in an airport line could be so life changing for Rachel, and for us.

Our current arrangement is not a long-term, sustainable solution. In Texas there is not much of a road map for adults with special needs. The absence of support services for adults with ASD is one of the reasons I become angry with the anti-vaccine lobby. They deplete a lot of oxygen from the room with their nonsense and false allegations, to the point where elected leaders, such as members of the Texas State Legislature, the Texas Congressional delegation, and the Office of the Governor and Lieutenant Governor, as well as other people in a position to make change could easily lose track of what families with ASD children really need—special services in school and after school, job placements, and programs for adults—in order to focus on vaccines.

I partly blame the anti-vaccine movement in America for why there are so few resources for adults and children with ASD. It's also why I consider the dozens of anti-vaccine organizations and websites, and the people who support such activities, to be both anti-child and anti-family. They place their own distorted ideologies ahead of the needs of children with ASD, and their families.

As it stands now, regarding Rachel, Ann and I are largely on our own.

· 12 ·

"Science Tikkun"

The anti-vaccine movement, especially in the United States and Europe, has been mostly successful in spite of the overwhelming evidence that vaccines do not cause autism, and in the face of overwhelming evidence for the genetic and epigenetic bases of ASD. Indeed, the anti-vaccine lobby has managed to persuade a generation of parents to opt their kids out of vaccinations despite the fact that they prevent the world's most dangerous childhood infections that kill hundreds of thousands of children annually. In its place the anti-vaxxers promote a narrative that has no scientific basis, nor even plausibility, while directly threatening the health and well-being of children. How did we allow things to get to this point?

In some countries, such as Pakistan or Afghanistan, anti-vaccine activities are driven by fear and ignorance fostered by the Taliban, which is intent on maintaining political dominance in a part of Central Asia at all costs, including the health of its children. It's disgusting and awful, but at some level we can begin to understand their political motives. In contrast, so far I'm not sure I truly understand the self-destructive motivations of the American anti-vaccine movement. It is a movement intent on placing America's children in harm's way for the sake of an ideology totally devoid of benefit.

In several of the 18 states that currently allow vaccine exemptions for nonmedical or philosophical reasons, the numbers of exemptions are rising dramatically. In the case of Texas, where there has been almost a 20-fold increase over the past decade, I attribute the rise to the fact that the anti-vaccine movement has been extremely well organized. Through both the movie *Vaxxed: From Cover-Up to Catastrophe*, and the rallies, marches, and lobbying activities of the political action committee, Texans for Vaccine Choice, a story has been concocted that is extremely compelling. The anti-vaccine lobby has made effective use of Twitter and other social media outlets.

Unfortunately, the Texas story, although compelling and convincing to those without a scientific background, also has no basis in reality. Instead it is a collection of fake news, half-truths, and conspiracy theories, which have been cleverly strung together to create a faux narrative. So how did it come to pass that such pseudoscience has been palmed off on the population of Texas, as well as many of the other 17 states that currently allow nonmedical vaccine exemptions?

Blaming Others

There's certainly no shortage of blame to go around. Vaccine policy is regulated at the state level, so that means there are 18 state legislatures that for some reason have remained susceptible and vulnerable to the misinformation put out by the anti-vaccine communities. But the anti-vaccine movement, especially in the United States, also has had a lot of help and from some unexpected sources. Certainly the media, even the mainstream media, has had an important role in perpetuating myths about vaccines and autism. On multiple major news outlets, including CNN, Fox News, MSNBC, and the major networks, I hear over and over again about the vaccine-autism "controversy," as though there really is a controversy about whether vaccines cause autism. By the way, they don't! To this day, most major television news outlets use almost every story I have ever seen about vaccine and autism to keep the door open about potential links and plausibility. They seldom pass up an opportunity to give a voice to prominent individuals with strong anti-vaccine views. For instance, I've heard both Tucker Carlson and Joe Scarborough conduct Fox News and MSNBC interviews, respectively, with a prominent anti-vaccine proponent (although my understanding is that Scarborough has since disavowed links between vaccines and autism) [1, 2]; I have watched a CNN anchor avoid challenging an anti-vaccine statement made by a leader of one of the nation's most prominent autism advocacy organizations; and I have heard a CBS field reporter speak about the drop in vaccine coverage in Minnesota as though it had some legitimate or rational basis.

Unfortunately, another and perhaps bigger problem, from my perspective, is the US government itself, which has been mostly silent about the rise in nonmedical exemptions and the dangers of not vaccinating children. So while I have not heard any US official actively promote anti-vaccine viewpoints, the leadership of the CDC, US Public Health Service, Department of Health and Human Services (DHHS), US National Institutes of Health, and the White House have nevertheless made few, if any, public statements refuting the *Vaxxed* movie or other incorrect assertions from the anti-vaccine community. I've been particularly frustrated by the office of the US Surgeon General, which in my opinion has been conspicuous in its absence on this issue. I think it's also important to point out that the silence from the US Surgeon General, DHHS, CDC, and White House cuts across the presidential tenure of both major parties. Yes, this is a problem in the Trump administration, but it was also true for the Obama, Bush, and Clinton administrations. We really need a strong and forceful US Surgeon General to warn about the dangers of withholding vaccines, to debunk specious links between vaccines and autism, and to actively tell people to vaccinate their children. I've been told that some of this government silence may be deliberate—that perhaps our officials don't want to provide undue attention to the anti-vaccine movement because they believe it's a fringe movement that will eventually go away. Maybe that was true in the years immediately following the publication of the 1998 *Lancet* article, but I think it's pretty clear that the anti-vaccine movement has since taken advantage of the silence and the vacuum to become well-funded and organized. I also believe that many Americans have come to believe that the American government's silence on this issue is somehow a tacit endorsement of anti-vaccine views.

An important reason for urging the media, state governments, and federal agencies to speak out in behalf of vaccines, while refuting the anti-vaccine community, is that they could make an important difference in convincing parents to vaccinate. From my experience, the majority of parents who choose to not vaccinate their kids are not actually deeply entrenched in their opposition. Instead, they have read something unsavory about vaccines on the Internet from one of the anti-vaccine websites, or they have been told something bad about vaccines by friends or relatives. For those parents, I have found that if you take the time to explain to them why vaccines are necessary and why they don't cause autism, or why their anti-vaccine neighbor, friend, spouse, boyfriend, or girlfriend is pushing misinformation, they begin to understand and agree to vaccinations.

However, I have also found that another 10–20 percent of parents harboring anti-vaccine views are indeed deeply dug in and have incorporated this mindset into their personal belief system, or even into their personal identity. In my experience, it's really tough, if not impossible, to reach those parents. As Cornelia Betsch, a German psychologist, has recently advised, "Forget about hardcore antivaxxers, but focus on those who haven't made up their minds" [3]. But for most parents we can make an enormous difference! The bottom line is that the stakes are high, and we need to find a way to better engage the public and parents about vaccines and autism.

Blaming Ourselves

In the end, I also blame us, meaning myself and the scientific community. I believe that we have been too reluctant to engage the public in a meaningful way in order to fight and counteract the false and misleading statements made on social media and the Internet, public rallies, and phony summits and documentaries.

According to the Pew Research Center in a study conducted in association with the American Association for the Advancement of Science (AAAS), as a profession, American scientists are not performing well in terms of public engagement. Their study found that while scientists support active engagement in public policy discussion in overwhelming numbers, the scientists themselves are not out there in the public eye. In a survey of 3,748 scientists, only about one-half have ever spoken with a reporter or science journalist about their research, while only 47 percent ever use social media to discuss their science. Only 24 percent have ever blogged about their science and research [4]. Not surprisingly, another study conducted by ResearchAmerica, an excellent policy and advocacy group based in Washington, DC, found in 2016 that an overwhelming majority—81 percent—of Americans could not name a living scientist, and after Stephen Hawking, Neil DeGrasse Tyson, and Bill Nye, the list dwindled quickly [5]. An older Research-America survey found that most Americans cannot name an institution that conducts biomedical research [6]. The Pew study also found that about one-half of scientists say that scientific findings are oversimplified in the media, while most (79 percent) believe that news reports "don't distinguish between well-founded and not well-founded scientific findings" [4].

I believe that the precipitous rise of the anti-vaccine movement has been enabled by a vacuum in public engagement by scientists. We're too focused on our grants and papers and have not allowed ourselves to devote time to public lectures, social media, blogs, print and electronic interviews, and other forms of public outreach. Similar reasons may also underlie the collapse of public support for aggressively addressing climate change and other timely scientific issues.

Public Engagement

A unique aspect of my scientific career is that I have from time to time made the effort to step away from the grants and papers. Since the early 2000s, I have had one foot in the laboratory focused on neglected disease vaccines and the other in the realm of public engagement. For instance, in order to persuade government leaders, donors, and the general public to become interested in NTDs such as schistosomiasis and Chagas disease

I have had to get out of the comfort zone of the laboratory to travel nationally and internationally in order to speak about these diseases and write for the public. This dual life is not an easy one for a number of reasons. First, my day job as a working scientist requires me to remain in Houston and keep up with the lab meetings and the discussions with our scientists, whereas my public engagement role generally means I need to be just about everywhere instead of Houston—Washington, DC; European capitals, especially London, Berlin, Paris, Amsterdam, and Geneva; Tokyo; and of course major cities in disease-endemic countries. In 2015 and 2016, I also served as US science envoy for the State Department and Obama White House, building science and vaccine diplomacy initiatives with Muslim-majority nations of the Middle East and North Africa. There is also the Texas component. I have served on two Texas governors' task forces on infectious diseases to combat Ebola and Zika virus in our state, and I have a meaningful relationship with the James A. Baker III Institute for Public Policy at Rice University, and occasionally also the Bush School for Public Policy at Texas A&M University. Overall, my public engagement activities require considerable travel, creating a dynamic tension between the two roles.

An added challenge is that public engagement is not usually considered a vital activity for a professor at an academic health center or university. These institutions depend on their faculty to generate revenue through clinical billing or research grants, and such public activities do not generally produce funds. Yet for someone like myself, committed to public engagement or aspiring to become a public intellectual, I have found that writing scientific papers and grant applications exclusively is seldom sufficient to persuade government leaders and policymakers to address a particular group of diseases or an approach to disease treatment and prevention. Instead, the information these papers and grants contain must be teased out and reorganized in formats more familiar to general audiences through writings and activities not considered traditional for an academic. They include op-eds and editorials; public lectures; testimonies before the US Congress, UK Parliament, and state legislatures; radio and TV interviews; speaking to journalists in the print media; having a presence on Twitter or other forms of social media; and even writing books for a general audience. Such books are perhaps the most demanding in terms of time commitment, but my first volume, *Forgotten People, Forgotten Diseases*, was absolutely essential to convey the health and economic impact of the NTDs, while *Blue Marble Health* appealed to the group of G20 leaders to also take on these diseases among their hidden poor [7, 8].

It also turns out there are not very many working scientists who juggle both science and public engagement responsibilities, probably and mostly owing to the enormous time commitments required by both endeavors. Revenue-generating grants and papers are considered paramount, whereas department chairs, deans, and even university presidents often care much less about public engagement. Moreover, there are no traditional metrics to assess the impact of public engagement when academic institutions seek to evaluate the productivity of their faculty. Recently, one brave soul attempted to address this situation by generating a science "Kardashian" impact that places your social media engagement through Twitter followers in the numerator and science citations in the denominator [9]. But I don't realistically see this measurement catching on within the academy.

Today, despite their importance, public engagement activities largely remain outside the traditional scope of academic health center activities, even though I believe we are now paying a steep price for our profession's lack of willingness to address public audiences. Indeed, I trace 15 or more years of essentially flat-line budgets for the US National Institutes of Health (NIH)—and currently threatened severe budget cuts—to the apathy or sometimes outright disdain of our scientists toward public activities. This long absence of budget increases at NIH has disproportionately affected young scientists, who now typically are not funded until they become midcareer investigators well into their 40s. I'm very concerned that we are losing a generation of young American scientists. This situation stands in stark contrast to nations such as China, Germany, and Singapore, which are now heavily investing in their young scientists. The future may belong to these nations.

I also believe the absence of public engagement is an important reason why an anti-vaccine movement based on pseudoscience or even outright falsehoods has been allowed to gain ascendancy in America.

PLOS and the *New York Times*

In addition to heading a tropical medicine school and vaccine institute in Texas, I also serve as founding editor in chief of *PLOS Neglected Tropical Diseases*, the first open access journal for tropical medicine. The open access concept was developed in the early twenty-first century and led to the formation of *PLOS*, which stands for the *Public Library of Science*. Essentially, anyone with a computer and Internet connection can download *PLOS* articles without worrying about a paywall that currently blocks access to most of the papers published in prestigious journals such as the *New England Journal of Medicine, JAMA* (*Journal of the American Medical Association*), and the *Lancet*. Today there are several prominent families of open access journals, including *PLOS*, *BioMed Central*, and *eLife*, among others. In addition, *Nature, Science*, and other traditional science publishers have now created new open access spin-off journals. This is an important trend that is revolutionizing science publishing and making important biomedical literature available to scientists across the planet.

Late in 2016, I began writing a series of articles, initially in one of our allied *PLOS* journals, *PLOS Medicine*, which in some ways represents the open access equivalent to high-profile general medical journals; and later in *PLOS Speaking of Medicine*, one of the best-known *PLOS* blog sites. The point of the articles was to warn about the events unfolding in Texas but also to assemble much of the salient literature justifying my assertions that vaccines did not cause autism.

The fact that each of these articles is open access means that they are widely available to journalists and can be made available easily on social media, including my very active Twitter account (@PeterHotez). It also means, of course, that the articles are also freely and widely available to the anti-vaccine community. One of the hallmarks of the anti-vaxxers is that they are very quick to pounce on articles that support vaccines and especially articles that refute their assertions and allegations. It's practically a given that whenever I write a piece that refutes a central anti-vaccine tenet linking either MMR vaccine or thimerosal to autism, or debunking the concept of spacing vaccines, I will receive a vigorous and shrill negative response on social media, especially Twitter, or in personal e-mails, or even phone calls. I tend to be quite an open and accessible individual—I do that deliberately in order to make myself available to students, residents, postdocs, and junior faculty—so reaching me through such mechanisms is relatively easy.

But nothing prepared me for the firestorm that resulted when I wrote an op-ed piece for the *New York Times* on February 8, 2017, titled "How the Anti-Vaxxers Are Winning" [10]. The piece had effects that were both good and bad. On the positive side, it alerted the general public to the anti-vaccine calamity brewing in Texas and the risk of it becoming nationwide. It highlighted an imminent measles risk to Texas and elsewhere in the United States, such as what then happened in Minnesota. It also succinctly summarized my evidence that vaccines do not cause autism and why it's not even plausible that vaccines cause autism. The article also attempted to debunk the *Vaxxed* movie and faux CDC conspiracies. In short, the *Times* piece provided a national and global stage to counteract the rising US anti-vaccine movement.

But there was also a dark side to how my op-ed was received. Previously, when it came to my public statements and writings about vaccines, the fact that I had a child (now adult) with autism and other severe mental disabilities kept me apart from the other well-known pro-vaccine voices, such as Seth Mnookin, author of *The Panic Virus* and Dr. Paul Offit at Children's Hospital of Philadelphia. While Seth and Paul endured many personal threats, for the most part I remained mostly beneath contempt. From time to time an anti-vaccine website would make some snarky and inappropriate remarks, and over the years I have received sporadic mean-spirited e-mails, but generally they had no effect on my work or public activities. After the *New York Times* article was published, however, the gloves really came off—at least through e-mails and social media. I went from being beneath contempt to becoming utterly contemptible.

Specifically, almost immediately after the op-ed was published I was subjected to a string of accusations from the anti-vaccine communities. Many of them alleged that I had become either a shill for industry or that I was making millions of dollars from my vaccines for neglected tropical diseases. The attacks also included a YouTube video alleging I was exaggerating the adverse health effects of measles, calling me "The Boy Who Cried Wolf," and some strange tirade pointing out that by living in a sanctuary city I was attempting to deliberately import measles into the United States in order to ignite an epidemic. In the end, the anti-vaccine communities faced a hard time making any accusation stick or sound credible. Although I wasn't exactly Teflon, one prominent anti-vaccine spokesperson actually issued a retraction and apology of sorts after I confronted him about his public statements.

Will the *New York Times* piece become an effective stopgap to halt or slow what I have termed an American neo-anti-vaccine movement? Probably not, but my goal in writing it was to become a prominent voice that could provide a reasonable alternative narrative for the autism parent community. My major message was that vaccines are safe and do not cause autism.

No single person will impede or stop the advance of what is rapidly becoming a very aggressive and organized initiative or movement. From their activities in the Somali community in the Twin Cities, and in Compton, California, it's also clear that the anti-vaxxers are not above predatory behavior in terms of their willingness to target vulnerable populations. However, as both a vaccine scientist and autism parent, my hope is that we can begin a long fight back to normalcy and scientific truthfulness in America. It's interesting to note that the steep rise of this neo-anti-vaccine movement roughly parallels other anti-science trends in America, including a sharp rebuke to climate change. The April 22, 2017, Earth Day march, when thousands of scientists rallied in Washington DC, and across the nation to protest anti-science threats across America, is perhaps the most tangible evidence that we might be entering a "new normal" when it comes to the need for American scientists to defend our values, principles, and practices.

"Science Tikkun"

I have also recently promoted the concept of "science tikkun" as an overarching framework for science diplomacy and public engagement [11]. The term "tikkun" comes from the phrase *tikkun olam*, referring to a Jewish obligation found in the Kabbalah and other ancient texts to repair the world [7]. I noted that the concept of *tikkun olam* reached its full expression in the sixteenth century, with the writings of Rabbi Isaac Luria. Luria was a Jewish mystic born in 1534 who lived mostly in areas of the Middle East occupied by the Ottoman Empire [11]. His concept of *tikkun olam* focused on repairing the world through good deeds and actions.

For me, it's of interest that such writings came to public attention around the time that some science historians indicate our modern concepts of experimental science first took root through the activities of Galileo Galilei and William Gilbert— two of the major figures identified by John Gribbin as among the first to use the modern experimental scientific method [11, 12]. Modern concepts of scientific experimentation and the concept of *tikkun olam* began contemporaneously. But since then the two fields diverged. "Science tikkun" seeks to unite the two concepts. Briefly, it represents a framework in which to think about public engagement in science. Through "science tikkun," scientists now have an added obligation to go beyond talking to themselves and instead to raise the profile of their findings and knowledge. We now need to go beyond the lab bench and incorporate into our activities public engagement by educating leaders in areas outside of our typical comfort zones. We need to take the time to educate leaders in all areas of business, religion, the media, the military, and government in order to help them to better understand science and scientific methods [11].

I believe that "science tikkun" will likely resonate well with young scientists. In my experience as a university professor and administrator, I regularly meet with students, postdocs, and junior faculty who crave more public engagement and involvement. My impression is that the commitment to public service by young scientists is at an all-time high, but they are frustrated by not having well-defined outlets for all this energy.

In the past, public engagement by scientists was seen as something unseemly or inappropriate and certainly not a proper or worthwhile activity. Now I believe we are paying the price for that inward looking attitude. It's one that created a vacuum for the anti-vaccine movement to grow and exert enormous influence to the point where measles has returned to America.

I'm not sure I really know how to put "the anti-vaccine genie back in the bottle," but I feel strongly that one piece of the solution is to fight back through public engagement by scientists in service of the public. It means we need to be more active in giving public lectures or town halls, reaching out to journalists, and being more active on social media. I appreciate that such activities might not be suitable for every scientist, but if we can have at least a substantial minority from our profession committed to "science tikkun" I believe we can go a long way to combating a rising tide of pseudoscience and ignorance.

First Steps: "What's Your Brand?"

Except during the summer, when things quiet down, I lecture to audiences about five times a month. My lectures are delivered through different forums, typically including medical or pediatric grand rounds or research seminars at academic health centers; classroom lectures; local, national, and international scientific meetings; but also community service organizations, breakfast clubs, and dinner events. Houston in particular is a very civic-minded city, and people enjoy attending public lectures. Whenever I speak to young audiences about "science tikkun" and public engagement, they seldom seem bored—they get it and are enthusiastic. My biggest problem is helping them get started on a path toward this goal. My professional life is now heavily imbued with "science tikkun," but I struggle to understand exactly how I got there and how to help others to create a road map.

There are not many formal mechanisms for career opportunities and development in scientific public engagement. They include the Science and Technology Fellowships offered by AAAS [13], which is an extraordinary program to place young scientists in government, but presumably this program cannot accommodate everyone. In addition, I have proposed the establishment of new government programs for scientific public engagement as a hedge against current and future anti-science activities in the United States and globally [11].

I also often meet individually with young people to advise them on career paths, including some committed to public engagement. One of my favorite things is to go to the white board with them to develop a 10-year plan. It's always amazing to me that I can speak with students, postdocs, and junior faculty and find out that no one has ever taken the time to ask them, "What does success look like for you 10 years down the road?" For many, this is a difficult question to answer, but one that I find immensely important for ensuring success, even if plans change midcourse (which is usually the case).

Another question I now routinely ask young scientists came about after I once heard a TV interview with Kobe Bryant, the former star basketball player from the Los Angeles Lakers. Kobe was being asked by a sports journalist about the imminent departure of Dwight Howard from the Lakers to become the center for the Houston Rockets (he subsequently joined the Rockets but then left to join the Atlanta Hawks, and then even moved on from there). Kobe said something that I thought was very wise, to the effect that Dwight had to do what was best for himself, his family, and his *brand*. It really hit me that for some, success as a scientist requires cultivating a brand. The brand includes the actual science of course, but also one's background, aspirations, gender, and sometimes cultural, political, or religious beliefs. It can represent the public face of a scientist. In my case, a Peter Hotez brand is a professor and laboratory investigator developing neglected disease vaccines, but also someone who through papers, op-eds, books, and lectures practices "science tikkun" and public engagement to provide access to essential vaccines and treatments for neglected diseases. Like my previous books, *Forgotten People, Forgotten Diseases* and *Blue Marble Health*, this book is part of the Peter Hotez brand. When young people visit me, I frequently ask them about their brand or try to help them begin the long process of developing one. It's an exercise many find both fun and meaningful.

Vaccine Science Diplomacy

For me, still another "science tikkun" activity is a concept I call "vaccine diplomacy" or "vaccine science diplomacy," in which I attempt to align my vaccine development activities with the shaping of US foreign policy. In a 2014 paper in *PLOS Neglected Tropical Diseases*, I defined these activities as follows: "*Vaccine diplomacy is the branch of global health diplomacy that relies on the use or delivery of vaccines, while vaccine science diplomacy is a unique hybrid of global health and science diplomacy.... *I use the term 'vaccine science diplomacy' narrowly to refer to the joint development of life-saving vaccines and related technologies, with the major actors typically scientists. Of particular interest, the scientists may be from two or more nations that often disagree ideologically or even from nations that are actively engaged in hostile actions" [14].

At our Texas Children's Center for Vaccine Development—a nonprofit university-based research institute making next-generation neglected disease vaccines—we have worked hard to build vaccines jointly with public sector institutions in Brazil, Mexico, and Malaysia. As mentioned earlier, in 2015–16, I served as a US science envoy focusing on vaccine science diplomacy and neglected disease vaccine development for the Middle East and North African region [15]. The position of US science envoy was established by President Obama and Secretary of State Hillary Clinton in 2009, in order to show a different face of America to the Muslim world. Recently, I noted that vaccine science diplomacy has an extraordinary Cold War legacy between the United States and the former Soviet Union, which led to the joint development of the oral polio vaccine and the smallpox eradication program [16]. I think vaccine diplomacy is an under-used concept in US foreign policy, but one that really puts our nation's best foot forward. For that reason I have proposed a robust expansion of our US Science Envoy program [11].

As the American anti-vaccine movement spreads internationally, I believe that we're going to once again need to tap a different type of vaccine diplomacy, this time through public engagement. We're seeing historically low levels of vaccine coverage in both western and eastern Europe. As of this writing, Romania is in the middle of a widespread measles outbreak, something that was unthinkable just a few years ago. We've allowed the anti-vaccine movement to go global, and now we will need international cooperation to reduce its impact. The stakes are high. As the anti-vaccine movement enters the world's low- and middle-income countries, we could face a dramatic reversal of the UN's Millennial Development Goals and see measles and other pediatric infections once considered relegated to the past become yet again major childhood killers.

In the meantime, here in the United States, we'll need "science tikkun" to begin chipping away at the damage done by the anti-vaccine lobby. Otherwise, measles outbreaks like the ones in California or among the Somali community in Minneapolis–St. Paul will be just the beginning of something far worse.

Epilogue

TALKING POINTS

In question-and-answer sessions following my public presentations, it's clear that pediatricians, primary care and family medicine physicians, and nurse practitioners are embattled. They are on the front lines, faced with the daunting task of convincing parents to vaccinate their children. Too often, parents are reading terrible things about vaccines on phony websites. They are hearing misinformation from their family and friends. In response, medical practitioners are being placed on the defensive about vaccines.

I recognize that explaining to parents, especially the ones who are truly cemented in their opposition, about the necessity of vaccines or of disregarding assertions that vaccines cause autism is no easy task. In a 2017 *New York Times* op-ed piece, the columnist Frank Bruni described the problem particularly well: "Over the past decade in particular, the internet and social media have changed the game. They speed people to like-minded warriors and give them the impression of broader company or sturdier validation than really exist. The fervor of those in the anti-vaccine movement exemplifies this" [1].

The big problem, of course, is that the Internet-fueled anti-vaccine movement has now translated into dangerous activities across the United States and now globally. Thousands of children are not receiving lifesaving vaccines, and we are facing imminent threats of measles outbreaks in the United States and Europe. Left unchecked, I believe it is only a matter of time before anti-vaccine fervor takes hold in major and highly populated low- and middle-income countries such as the BRICS nations (Brazil, Russia, India, China, and South Africa) or in Bangladesh, Indonesia, and Nigeria. The movement will begin with the middle and upper classes, who will read the phony claims and anti-science rhetoric on the Internet, but then quickly spill over to those who live in poverty.

General Talking Points

Aside from reaching government leaders and elected officials and persuading them to close vaccine loopholes such as non-medical or philosophical belief exemptions, it will largely fall to health-care providers to explain to parents the need for vaccines and why they will not cause autism in their children.

To summarize from this book, here are a few general talking points for health practitioners on the front lines:

- *Childhood vaccines save lives.* Before the creation of Gavi, the Vaccine Alliance, it's estimated that more than 12 million children died every year before the age of five. Through widespread vaccination against more than a dozen diseases, including diphtheria, pertussis, tetanus, Hib, polio, rotavirus, pneumococcal pneumonia, measles, mumps, rubella, and others, that number has been cut to about 4 million childhood deaths every year. The only thing protecting your child from these diseases is scheduled vaccinations. Diseases such as measles are not benign illnesses. In recent measles outbreaks in California and Minnesota, dozens of children required hospitalization and could have died. After smallpox was eradicated in the late 1970s and until Gavi came along, measles was the single leading killer of children globally. Indeed, before measles vaccine was introduced in the United States in the early 1960s, around 500 children died annually, while 50,000 required hospitalization [2]. Many of those hospitalized were permanently neurologically impaired. Moreover, new information from previous California outbreaks shows that the severe and long-term permanent brain and neurologic complication of measles known as SSPE is far more common than we previously realized. These points are important because one of the rising assertions from the anti-vaccine groups is that measles is nothing more than a rash and fever. Nothing could be further than the truth—it is a great killer of children, and the only way to protect a child against measles is by vaccination.

- *Childhood vaccines do not cause autism, plain and simple.* This truth has been shown over and over again in clinical (epidemiological) studies involving more than one million children across the globe. They represent studies published in the medical profession's finest and most rigorous biomedical journals, including the *New England Journal of Medicine, JAMA, Lancet,* and *PLOS Medicine.* The studies show that measles-mumps-rubella vaccine does not cause autism; thimerosal-containing vaccines do not cause autism; and administering vaccines closely together in time does not cause autism. Alum in vaccines does not cause autism. Such studies are summarized in chapter 8 of this book and also the *Public Library of Science* (*PLOS*), which is freely accessible on the Web [3].

- *The causes of autism are something other than vaccines.* The science further provides overwhelming evidence that the changes in the brains of children with autism begin prenatally, well before children receive their vaccinations. So far, at least 65 genes have been identified that result in these brain alterations. While you might have heard that some children become autistic after receiving their vaccines between one and two years of age, the science shows that while children often first display overtly autistic behaviors at that time, or even begin regressing in language, speech, and communication between those ages, we can now show by MRI that those children had brain changes far earlier—when they were about six months old. In turn, those children had changes in their brains even when they were still developing as a fetus. This information is summarized in chapter 9 of this book and is also available on a Baylor College of Medicine blog that I wrote in 2017 [4].

- *There is an abundance of deliberately misleading information on the Internet.* According to a recent *Time* magazine article, there are now 480 major anti-vaccine websites [5]. To respond to such false claims, many of the points raised above can be addressed by going to the "vaccine hesitancy" section of the public policy webpage found at our National School of Tropical Medicine, Baylor College of Medicine website [6], or by going to the CDC website on vaccine safety [7]. The World Health Organization also has a website on this topic [8], while the American Academy of Pediatrics maintains a helpful website for health-care providers on how to speak with vaccine-hesitant parents or guardians [9].

Specific Talking Points for Special Concerns

In addition to the general points highlighted above, vaccine-hesitant parents or anti-vaccine groups often raise objections that go well beyond concerns about autism. Here are a few of them:

- *Myth: Mandatory vaccination is part of a conspiracy.* There are a fair number of conspiracy theories out there related to vaccines. Generally they involve the US and foreign governments, the CDC, multinational pharmaceutical companies, or some combination of the three. The movie *Vaxxed: From Cover-Up to Catastrophe* is deeply imbued with conspiracy theories, including an overarching one that the CDC is involved in regarding squashing a whistleblower. A number of websites claim the CDC or the US government is in the pockets of Big Pharma. One of the hazards of trying to persuade someone that there is no conspiracy is that you risk making that individual think that you yourself might be part of the conspiracy. The truth, of course, is that there is no conspiracy. Anyone who has worked with the CDC—or any part of the government bureaucracy—realizes pretty quickly that, even if it wanted to cover something up, the concealment would last about one afternoon, if that. Federal agencies in the United States are simply not organized for keeping secrets. A major problem, and one that I point out in this book, is that US government leaders involved in public health have been mostly silent about vaccines. We urgently need a strong and independent US Surgeon General, as well as other high-ranking individuals at the Department of Health and Human Services, to speak out forcefully about the importance of vaccinating children and explain why vaccines are safe.

- *Myth: The diseases are gone, and we no longer need vaccines.* Nothing could be further from the truth. We are now seeing the return of measles to the United States and Europe, as well as mumps, pertussis, and several others. These are diseases that kill or cause permanent brain and neurologic injury. Worldwide, approximately 750,000 children under the age of five died in 2015 from vaccine-preventable diseases such as pneumococcal pneumonia, rotaviral enteritis, measles, Hib, pertussis, tetanus, and diphtheria [10].

- *Myth: More children in the United States die from vaccines than from the diseases they prevent.* This point is a corollary or follows from the previous one. We have done a good job in preventing deaths from diseases for which we now have vaccines. But only if we continue vaccinating. Regarding the actual assertion about more people dying from vaccines than the diseases they prevent, it is a false one. As explained in chapter 10, the chances of experiencing a serious adverse event from an immunization are about the same as being struck by lightning. Here's another way to look at the data: According to CDC mortality data, approximately 2.63 million Americans died in the year 2014. These numbers include 4,605 people who died from influenza; 50,622 who died from pneumonia, which presumably includes a high percentage of deaths resulting from pneumococcal pneumonia; 9,773 from "certain other intestinal infections," of which possibly some died from rotaviral enteritis; 43 from meningococcal infection; and 14 from whooping cough. In total this equates to around 65,000 deaths. If we focus only on children, then approximately 32,000 American children under the age of 15 died in 2014. These deaths include 122 from influenza, 271 from pneumonia, 248 from "certain other intestinal infections," 8 from meningococcal infection, and 12 from whooping cough. In all, this number represents 661 childhood deaths [11]. According to Politifact, 122 deaths were reported to the Vaccine Adverse Event Reporting System in 2014 [12]. But this number includes deaths from causes totally un-related to receiving the actual vaccine. Essentially any death for whatever reason that occurs around the time of vaccination can be reported to VAERS. So the actual num-ber of deaths from vaccines annually is almost certainly under 100, and probably far less than that. Thus, the asser-tion is false.

- *Myth: Our body's own "natural" immunity is adequate.* Almost a million children who rely on their "natural" im-mune system die annually from vaccine-preventable dis-eases. Before Gavi, that number was several times higher. Another point often raised is the concern about "over-whelming" the immune system with vaccines. Again, there is no evidence for this belief, and in fact a newborn's developing immune system receives many, and likely hun-dreds, of new antigens every day through lymphoid tissue found in its lungs and intestines. As I have shown in chap-ter 10, there is also no proven link between vaccines and autoimmune or other immunological disorders.

- *Concern about vaccine ingredients.* Reading the package insert of a vaccine reveals the presence of a number of ex-cipients (inert substances that form a vehicle for the drug) that cause concern among some parents. It's important to point out that the FDA mandates showing that each of these excipients is required to maintain the stability of the vaccine or to ensure its safety and effectiveness. I can personally say that when we're advancing one of our neglected disease vaccines to clinical trials and submitting investigational new drug filings to the FDA, we have to justify and prove the safety and necessity of each component. Through rigorous and carefully monitored phase 1, 2, and 3 clinical trials, the FDA requires extensive safety testing of vaccines, a process that can easily take up to a decade. Even after a vaccine is introduced, it continues to be carefully monitored through post-licensure studies, and then there is the Vaccine Adverse Event Reporting System. In other words, there are multiple safety nets in place to follow the tracks of every vaccine, and even every lot of vaccine used in the United States.

- *Other issues.* Dr. Tara Smith at Kent State University has also identified some of the same issues I have highlighted above. She points to additional myths, which include the idea that "diseases have declined on their own due to improved hygiene and sanitation" rather than vaccines [13]. There is no question that higher living standards have reduced infectious disease burdens globally, but the evidence is overwhelming that vaccines have done the most to bring down ancient childhood scourges. For example, according to the Global Burden of Disease Study, almost one million people died annually from measles in 1990, and that number was reduced to around 600,000 by 2000 through WHO's Expanded Programme on Immunization [14]. However, now through Gavi, the Vaccine Alliance, fewer than 70,000 people die annually from measles [14]. Such dramatic declines could only be accounted for through expanded use of the measles or MMR vaccine. Dr. Smith also highlights an often-heard comment that vaccines haven't been tested in randomized clinical trials [13], which is also untrue. In my conversations with prominent anti-vaccine activists, I've learned that they now want to see a massively powered study that compares autism rates among children randomized to either receive their full complement of childhood vaccines versus no vaccines at all. I point out that it would be unethical to conduct such a trial given that vaccines are lifesaving and there is no evidence that vaccines cause autism.

Clearly, the talking points provided above cannot address all of the concerns raised by vaccine-hesitant parents. But my hope is that the contents of this book will overall provide assurances to parents and health-care providers about the safety of vaccines and a detailed account of why vaccines do *not* cause autism, the cornerstone of today's anti-vaccine movement. There are enormous consequences to not vaccinating children in the United States, Europe, and globally. I believe there is great risk that today's anti-vaccine activities could snowball into something much larger and possibly endanger the next generation of the world's children. Although we are living in a scary time, there is still much we can do to reduce the global risk of emerging and childhood infectious diseases.

References

Chapter 1. Family Interrupted

1. Hotez PJ (2014) The medical biochemistry of poverty and neglect. Mol Med 20 (Suppl 1): S31–36.
2. Keating C (2017) Kenneth Warren and the Great Neglected Diseases of Mankind Programme: The transformation of geographical medicine in the US and beyond. Springer.
3. Stoll NR (1962) On endemic hookworm, where do we stand today? Exp Parasitol 12: 241–52.
4. Hotez PJ, Bottazzi ME, Strych U (2016) New vaccines for the world's poorest people. Annu Rev Med 67: 405–17.
5. Wakefield AJ, Murch SH, Anthony A, Linnell J, Casson DM, Malik M, Berelowitz M, et al. (1998) Ileal-lymphoid-nodular hyperplasia, nonspecific colitis, and pervasive developmental disorder in children. Lancet 351(9103): 637–41. Erratum in: Lancet 2004 363(9411): 750. Retraction in: Lancet 2010 375(9713): 445.
6. Bernard S, Enayati A, Redwood L, Roger H, Binstock T (2001) Autism: A novel form of mercury poisoning. Med Hypotheses 56(4): 462–71.

Chapter 2. Saving Lives with Vaccines

1. Briere EC, Rubin L, Moro PL, Cohn A, Clark T, Messonnier N; Division of Bacterial Diseases, National Center for Immunization and Respiratory Diseases, CDC (2014). Prevention and control of *Haemophilus influenzae* type b disease: Recommendations of the advisory committee on immunization practices (ACIP). MMWR Recomm Rep. 2014 Feb 28;63(RR-01): 1–14. https://www.cdc.gov/mmwr/preview/mmwrhtml/rr6301a1.htm.
2. https://www.cdc.gov/hi-disease/vaccination.html.

3. Anderson P, Peter G, Johnston RB Jr, Wetterlow LH, Smith DH (1972) Immunization of humans with polyribophosphate, the capsular antigen of *Hemophilus influenza*, type b. J Clin Invest 51(1): 39–44.

4. Schneerson R, Barrera O, Sutton A, Robbins JB (1980) Preparation, characterization, and immunogenicity of *Haemophilus influenzae* type b polysaccharide-protein conjugates. J Exp Med 152(2): 361–76.

5. McLean HQ, Fiebelkorn AP, Temte JL, Wallace GS; Centers for Disease Control and Prevention (2013) Prevention of measles, rubella, congenital rubella syndrome, and mumps, 2013: summary recommendations of the Advisory Committee on Immunization Practices (ACIP). MMWR Recomm Rep. 62(RR-04): 1–34.

6. https://www.cdc.gov/tetanus/surveillance.html.

7. https://www.cdc.gov/pertussis/images/incidence-graph.png.

8. https://www.cdc.gov/diphtheria/about/index.html.

9. https://www.cdc.gov/rotavirus/surveillance.html.

10. Schwartz JL, Mahmoud A (2014) A half-century of prevention—The Advisory Committee on Immunization Practices. N Engl J Med 371: 1953–56.

11. https://www.cdc.gov/vaccines/parents/diseases/child/index.html.

12. Rodewald LE, Orenstein WA, Hinman AR, Schuchat A (2013) Immunization in the United States. In: Vaccines, eds. Plotkin SA, Orenstein WA, Offit PA. 6th ed., Elsevier, pp. 1310–33.

13. Hotez PJ (2017) Science and America's greatness. Sci Am April 7. https://blogs.scientificamerican.com/guest-blog/science-and -americas-greatness.

14. Henderson DA (2009) Smallpox: The death of a disease. Prometheus Books.

15. https://www.washingtonpost.com/local/obituaries/da-henderson-disease -detective-who-eradicated-smallpox-dies-at-87/2016/08/20/b270406e -63dd-11e6-96c0-37533479f3f5_story.html?utm_term=.d219a7a718a8.

16. Hotez PJ (2014) "Vaccine diplomacy": Historical perspectives and future directions. PLOS Negl Trop Dis 8(6): e2808.

17. Guyer B, Atangana S (1977) A programme of multiple-antigen childhood immunization in Yaounde, Cameroon: First-year evaluation, 1975–1976. Bull World Health Organ 55(5): 633–42.

18. http://www.vaccinationcouncil.org/2009/06/18/the-childrens-vaccine -initiative-an-open-window-upon-global-vaccination-strategies.

19. Muraskin W (1998) The politics of international health: The Children's Vaccine Initiative and the struggle to develop vaccines for the third world. State University of New York Press.

20. http://www.gavi.org/about/mission.

21. http://www.gavi.org/about/mission/facts-and-figures.

22. GBD 2015 Mortality and Causes of Death Collaborators (2016) Global, regional, and national life expectancy, all-cause mortality, and cause-specific mortality for the 249 causes of death, 1980–2015: A systematic analysis for the Global Burden of Disease Study 2015. Lancet 388: 1459–544.

Chapter 3. A Mostly Noncompliant Little Girl

1. Hazlett HC, Gu H, Munsell BC, Kim SH, Styner M, Wolff JJ, Elison JT, et al. (2017) Early brain development in infants at high risk for autism spectrum disorder. Nature 542: 348–51.

2. Emerson RW, Adams C, Nishino T, Hazlett HC, Wolff JJ, et al (2017) Functional neuroimaging of high-risk 6-month-old infants predicts a diagnosis of autism at 24 months of age. Sci Translational Med 9(393): eaag2882.

Chapter 4. Derailment

1. http://sitn.hms.harvard.edu/flash/special-edition-on-infectious-disease/ 2014/the-fight-over-inoculation-during-the-1721-boston-smallpox -epidemic.

2. Poland GA, Jacobson RM (2011) The age-old struggle against the anti-vaccinationists. N Engl J Med 364: 97–99.

3. Eggers C (1976) Autistic syndrome (Kanner) and vaccination against smallpox (author's transl). Klin Padiatr 188(2): 172–80. German.

4. Wakefield AJ, Murch SH, Anthony A, Linnell J, Casson DM, Malik M, Berelowitz M, et al. (1998) Ileal-lymphoid-nodular hyperplasia, non-specific colitis, and pervasive developmental disorder in children. Lancet 351(9103): 637–41. Erratum in: Lancet 2004 363(9411): 750. Retraction in: Lancet 2010 375(9713): 445.

5. Godlee F, Smith J, Marcovitch H (2011) Wakefield's article linking MMR vaccine and autism was fraudulent. BMJ 342: c7452.

6. Deer B (2011) How the case against the MMR vaccine was fixed. BMJ 342: c5347. doi: 10.1136/bmj.c5347.

7. Deer B (2011) Secrets of the MMR scare: How the vaccine crisis was meant to make money. BMJ 342: c5258. doi: 10.1136/bmj.c5258.

8. Deer B (2011) Secrets of the MMR scare: The *Lancet*'s two days to bury bad news. BMJ 342: c7001. doi: 10.1136/bmj.c7001.

9. Deer B (2011) Pathology reports solve "new bowel disease" riddle. BMJ 343: d6823. doi: 10.1136/bmj.d6823.

10. Deer B (2011) More secrets of the MMR scare: Who saw the "histological findings"? BMJ 343: d7892. doi: 10.1136/bmj.d7892.

11. Chatterjee A (2013) The controversy that will not go away: Vaccines and autism. In: Vaccinophobia and vaccine controversies of the 21st century, ed. Chatterjee A. Springer, pp. 189–91.

12. https://www.theguardian.com/uk-news/2016/mar/11/sudden-increase -uk-measles-cases-warning-mmr-vaccination.

13. https://ecdc.europa.eu/en/news-events/epidemiological-update-measles -monitoring-european-outbreaks-22-june-2017.

14. http://www.npr.org/sections/goatsandsoda/2017/04/07/522867040/ as-measles-surges-in-europe-officials-brace-for-a-rough-year.

15. Durrheim DN, Crowcroft NS, Strebel PM (2014) Measles: The epidemiol-ogy of elimination. Vaccine 32: 6880–83. pmid:25444814.

16. Bernard S, Enayati A, Redwood L, Roger H, Binstock T (2001) Autism: A novel form of mercury poisoning. Med Hypotheses 56(4): 462–71.

17. Baker JP (2008) Mercury, vaccines, and autism: One controversy, three histories. Am J Publ Health 98(2): 244–53.

18. Kennedy RF, Hyman M, Herbert MR, Posey B, eds. Thimerosal: Let the science speak; The evidence supporting the immediate removal of mercury—a known neurotoxin—from vaccines. Skyhorse Publishing.

19. https://www.fda.gov/BiologicsBloodVaccines/SafetyAvailability/Vaccine Safety/UCM096228.

20. https://www.cdc.gov/vaccinesafety/concerns/thimerosal/timeline.html.

21. Sears RW (2011) The vaccine book: Making the right decision for your child. Sears Parenting Library.

22. Offit PA, Moser CA (2009) The problem with Dr. Bob's alternative vaccine schedule. Pediatrics 123(1): e164–69.

23. Gerber JS, Offit PA (2009) Vaccines and autism: A tale of shifting hypothe-ses. Clin Infect Dis 48(4): 456–61.

24. https://sciencebasedmedicine.org/jenny-mccarthy-jim-carrey-and-green -our-vaccines-anti-vaccine-not-pro-safe-vaccine.

25. McKee AS, Marrack P (2017) Old and new adjuvants. Curr Opin Immunol 47: 44–51.

26. https://www.fda.gov/BiologicsBloodVaccines/SafetyAvailability/Vaccine Safety/ucm187810.htm.

27. Hotez PJ, Strych U, Lustigman S, Bottazzi ME (2016) Human anthelminthic vaccines: Rationale and challenges. Vaccine 34(30): 3549–55.

28. Dyer O (2017) Canadian researchers whose studies questioned vaccine safety face second retraction. BMJ 359: j4904.

Chapter 5. Like Rome during the Roman Empire

1. Collier P (2007) The bottom billion: Why the poorest countries are failing and what can be done about it. Oxford University Press.

2. Molyneux DH, Hotez PJ, Fenwick A (2005) "Rapid-impact interventions": How a policy of integrated control for Africa's neglected tropical diseases could benefit the poor. PLOS Med 2(11): e336.

3. Hotez PJ, Molyneux DH, Fenwick A, Ottesen E, Ehrlich Sachs S, Sachs JD (2006) Incorporating a rapid-impact package for neglected tropical diseases with programs for HIV/AIDS, tuberculosis, and malaria. PLOS Med 3(5): e102.

4. Hotez PJ, Molyneux DH, Fenwick A, Kumaresan J, Sachs SE, Sachs JD, Savioli L (2007) Control of neglected tropical diseases. N Engl J Med 357(10): 1018–27.

5. Hotez PJ (2013) Forgotten people, forgotten diseases: The neglected tropical diseases and their impact on global health and development. ASM Press.

6. Grieder E (2013) Big, hot, cheap, and right: What America can learn from the strange genius of Texas. PublicAffairs.

7. Hotez PJ (2016) Blue marble health: An innovative plan to fight diseases of the poor amid wealth. Johns Hopkins University Press.

Chapter 6. The British Invasion

1. https://ecdc.europa.eu/en/news-events/epidemiological-update-measles-monitoring-european-outbreaks-7-july-2017.

2. http://www.nobelprize.org/nobel_prizes/medicine/laureates/1954/enders-bio.html.

3. Hotez PJ (2016) Texas and its measles epidemics. PLOS Med 13(10): e1002153. https://doi.org/10.1371/journal.pmed.1002153.

4. Orenstein WA, Papania MJ, Wharton ME (2004) Measles elimination in the United States. J Infect Dis 189 (Suppl 1): S1–3. pmid:15106120.

5. Strebel PM, Papania MJ, Fiebelkorn AP, Halsey NA (2013) Measles vaccine. In: Vaccines, eds. Plotkin, SA, Orenstein WA, Offit PA. 6th ed., Elsevier, pp. 352–87.

6. https://www.youtube.com/watch?v=IG5T_lE0wp8.

7. Offit PA (2007) Vaccinated: One man's quest to defeat the world's deadliest diseases. Smithsonian Books.

8. https://www.cdc.gov/measles/about/history.html.

9. Centers for Disease Control and Prevention (CDC) (2008) Measles: United States, January 1–April 25, 2008. MMWR Morb Mortal Wkly Rep 57(18): 494–98.

10. http://www.ncsl.org/research/health/school-immunization-exemption -state-laws.aspx.

11. Richards JL, Wagenaar BH, Van Otterloo J, Gondalia R, Atwell JE, Kleinbaum DG, Salmon DA, et al. (2013) Nonmedical exemptions to immunization requirements in California: A 16-year longitudinal analysis of trends and associated community factors. Vaccine 31(29): 3009–13.

12. McNutt LA, Desemone C, DeNicola E, El Chebib H, Nadeau JA, Bednarczyk RA, Shaw J (2016) Affluence as a predictor of vaccine refusal and underimmunization in California private kindergartens. Vaccine 34(14): 1733–38.

13. Zipprich J, Winter K, Hacker J, Xia D, Watt J, Harriman K; Centers for Disease Control and Prevention (CDC) (2015) Measles outbreak: California, December 2014–February 2015. MMWR Morb Mortal Wkly Rep. 64(6): 153–54.

14. http://blog.sfgate.com/stew/2015/02/04/jon-stewart-goes-after -marin-county-over-measles-outbreak.

15. Delamater PL, Leslie TF, Yang YT (2016) A spatiotemporal analysis of non-medical exemptions from vaccination: California schools before and after SB 277. Soc Sci Med 168: 230–38.

16. Offit P (2017) Who's cheating California's tough new vaccine system? Daily Beast, September 2. http://www.thedailybeast.com/whos-cheating -californias-tough-new-vaccine-system.

17. Opel DJ, Schwartz JL, Omer SB, Silverman R, Duchin J, Kodish E, Diekema DS, et al. (2017) Achieving an optimal childhood vaccine policy. JAMA Pediatrics [Epub ahead of print].

18. Wendorf KA, Winter K, Zipprich J, Schechter R, Hacker JK, Preas C, Cherry JD, et al. (2017) Subacute sclerosing panencephalitis: The devastating measles complication that might be more common than previ-

ously estimated. Clin Infect Dis. doi: 10.1093/cid/cix302 [Epub ahead of print].

19. https://www.washingtonpost.com/national/health-science/anti-vaccine -activists-spark-a-states-worst-measles-outbreak-in-decades/2017/05/04/ a1fac952-2f39-11e7-9dec-764dc781686f_story.html?tid=ss_tw&utm_term= .16738fe757ef.

20. Clemmons NS, Wallace GS, Patel M, Gastañaduy PA (2017) Incidence of measles in the United States, 2001–2015. JAMA 318(13): 1279–81.

21. Sun LH (2017) Failure to vaccinate is likely driver of US measles outbreaks, report says. Washington Post, October 3. https://www.washingtonpost .com/news/to-your-health/wp/2017/10/03/failure-to-vaccinate-is-likely -driver-of-u-s-measles-outbreaks-report-says/?utm_term=.204357e9ccf6.

22. Lo NC, Hotez PJ (2017) Public health and economic consequences of vaccine hesitancy for measles in the United States. JAMA Pediatr 171(9): 887–92.

23. https://www.texastribune.org/2016/07/14/see-studnet-vaccine-exemptions -school.

24. https://www.washingtonpost.com/national/health-science/trump -energizes-the-anti-vaccine-movement-in-texas/2017/02/20/795bd3ae -ef08-11e6-b4ff-ac2cf509efe5_story.html?utm_term=.52ad2e8751e3.

25. http://scienceblogs.com/insolence/2016/05/25/andrew-wakefield-and-del -bigtree-privileged-white-males-harming-african-americans-with-anti vaccine-misinformation.

26. https://www.statnews.com/2016/04/01/vaxxed-autism-movie-review.

27. http://vaxxedthemovie.com/vaxxed-nation-tour.

28. http://www.npr.org/2013/09/01/217746942/texas-megachurch-at-center-of -measles-outbreak.

29. https://twitter.com/realdonaldtrump/status/449525268529815552?lang=en.

30. http://fortune.com/2017/02/16/donald-trump-autism-vaccines.

31. http://www.cnn.com/2017/01/10/politics/robert-f-kennedy-jr-donald -trump-vaccine-commission.

32. Larson HJ, de Figueiredo A, Xiahong Z, Schulz WS, Verger P, Johnston IG, Cook AR, et al. (2016) The state of vaccine confidence 2016: Global insights through a 67-country survey. EBioMedicine 12: 295–301.

33. Alves Barbieri CL, Couto MT (2015) Decision making on childhood vacci-nation by highly educated parents. Rev Saude Publica 49: 18.

34. Hotez PJ (2017) Will an American-led anti-vaccine movement subvert global health? Sci Am, March 3. https://blogs.scientificamerican.com/

guest-blog/will-an-american-led-anti-vaccine-movement-subvert-global
-health.

Chapter 7. Montrose

1. Szalavitz M (2016) Autism: It's different in girls. Sci Am March 1.
   https://www.scientificamerican.com/article/autism-it-s-different-in-girls.
2. http://www.cam.ac.uk/research/news/girls-with-anorexia-have-elevated
   -autistic-traits.

Chapter 8. Vaccines Don't Cause Autism

1. Hotez P (2017) The "Why vaccines don't cause autism" papers. PLOS
   Speaking of Medicine, January 20. http://blogs.plos.org/speakingof
   medicine/2017/01/20/the-why-vaccines-dont-cause-autism-papers.
2. American Academy of Pediatrics (2013) Vaccine safety: Examine the
   evidence. https://www.aap.org/en-us/Documents/immunization_vaccine_
   studies.pdf.
3. Madsen KM, Hviid A, Vestergaard M, Schendel D, Wohlfahrt J, Thorsen
   P, Olsen J, et al. (2002) A population-based study of measles, mumps, and
   rubella vaccination and autism. N Engl J Med 347: 1477–82.
4. Smeeth L, Cook C, Fombonne E, Heavey L, Rodrigues L, Smith PG, Hall
   AJ (2004) MMR vaccination and pervasive developmental disorders:
   A case-control study. Lancet 364: 963–69.
5. D'Souza Y, Fombonne E, Ward BJ (2006) No evidence of persisting measles virus in peripheral blood mononuclear cells from children with autism
   spectrum disorder. Pediatrics 118: 1664–75.
6. Jain A, Marshall J, Buikema A, Bancroft T, Kelly JP, Newschaffer CJ (2015)
   Autism occurrence by MMR vaccine status among US children with older
   siblings with and without autism. JAMA 313(15): 1534–40.
7. Uno Y, Uchiyama T, Kurosawa M, Aleksic B, Ozaki N (2015) Early exposure to the combined measles-mumps-rubella vaccine and thimerosal-
   containing vaccines and risk of autism spectrum disorder. Vaccine 33(21):
   2511–16.
8. Taylor LE, Swerdfeger AL, Eslick GD (2014) Vaccines are not associated
   with autism: An evidence-based meta-analysis of case-control and cohort
   studies. Vaccine 32(29): 3623–29.
9. https://www.cdc.gov/vaccinesafety/concerns/thimerosal/index.html.

10. https://www.cdc.gov/mmwr/volumes/65/rr/rr6505a1.htm.

11. Schechter R, Grether JK (2008) Continuing increases in autism reported to California's Developmental Services System. Arch Gen Psychiatry 65(1): 19–24.

12. Hviid A, Stellfeld M, Wholfahrt J, Melbye M (2003) Association between thimerosal-containing vaccine and autism. JAMA 290: 1763–66.

13. Madsen K, Lauritsen MB, Pedersen CB, Thorsen P, Plesner A-M, Andersen PH, Mortensen PB (2003) Thimerosal and the occurrence of autism: Negative ecological evidence from Danish population-based data. Pediatrics 112: 604–6.

14. English C, Yutuc V, Ferrier C, Sackett GP, Marti CN, Young K, Hewitson L, et al. (2015) Administration of thimerosal-containing vaccines to infant rhesus macaques does not result in autism-like behavior or neuropathology. Proc Natl Acad Sci USA 112(40): 12498–503.

15. Zerbo O, Qian Y, Yoshida C, Fireman BH, Klein NP, Croen LA (2017) Association between influenza infection and vaccination during pregnancy and risk of autism spectrum disorder. JAMA Pediatr 171(1): e163609.

16. http://katlynfoxfoundation.com.

17. Garcon N, Friede M (2018) Evolution of adjuvants across the centuries. In: Plotkin's vaccines, eds. Plotkin SA, Orenstein WA, Offit PA, Edwards KM. 7th ed., Elsevier, pp. 61–75.

18. http://www.chop.edu/centers-programs/vaccine-education-center/vaccine-ingredients/aluminum.

Chapter 9. What Does Cause Autism?

1. https://www.cdc.gov/ncbddd/autism/signs.html.

2. Ozonoff S, Heung K, Byrd R, Hansen R, Hertz-Picciotto I (2008) The onset of autism: Patterns of emergence in the first years of life. Autism Res 1(6): 320–28.

3. Volkmar FR, Cohen DJ (1989) Disintegrative disorder or "late onset" autism. J Child Psychol 30(5): 717–24.

4. Kobayashi R, Murata T (1998) Setback phenomenon in autism and long-term prognosis. Acta Psychiatrica Scandinavica 98(4): 296–303.

5. GBD 2015 Disease and Injury Incidence and Prevalence Collaborators (2016) Global, regional, and national incidence, prevalence and years lived with disability for 310 diseases and injuries, 1990–2015: A systematic analysis for the Global Burden of Disease Study 2015. Lancet 388: 1545–602.

6. Kanner L (1946) Irrelevant and metaphorical language in early infantile autism. Am J Psychiatry 103(2): 242–46.

7. Bailey A, Luthert P, Bolton P, Le Couteur A, Rutter M, Harding B (1993) Autism and megalencephaly. Lancet 341(8854): 1225–26.

8. Davidovitch M, Patterson B, Gartside P (1996) Head circumference measurements in children with autism. J Child Neurol 11(5): 389–93.

9. Lainhart JE, Piven J, Wzorek M, Landa R, Santangelo SL, Coon H, Folstein SE (1997) Macrocephaly in children and adults with autism. J Am Acad Child Adolesc Psychiatry 36(2): 282–90.

10. Klein S, Sharifi-Hannauer P, Martinez-Agosto JA (2013) Macrocephaly as a clinical indicator of genetic subtypes in autism. Autism Research 6(1): 51–56.

11. Courchesne E, Carper R, Akshoomoff N (2003) Evidence of brain overgrowth in the first year of life in autism. JAMA 290(3): 337–44.

12. Hotez PJ (2017) Autism spectrum disorder: If not vaccines, then what? From the Labs (blog), February 24. https://fromthelabs.bcm.edu/2017/02/24/autism-spectrum-disorder-if-not-vaccines-then-what.

13. Hazlett HC, Gu H, Munsell BC, Kim SH, Styner M, Wolff JJ, ... Piven J, et al. (2017) Early brain development in infants at high risk for autism spectrum disorder. Nature 542: 348–51.

14. Emerson RW, Adams C, Nishino T, Hazlett HC, Wolff JJ, Zwaigenbaum L, ... Piven J (2017) Functional neuroimaging of high-risk 6-month-old infants predicts a diagnosis of autism at 24 months of age. Sci Translational Med 9(393): eaag2882.

15. https://www.cdc.gov/vaccines/schedules/hcp/imz/child-adolescent.html.

16. Stoner R, Chow ML, Boyle MP, Sunkin S, Mouton PR, Roy S, ... Courchesne E (2014) Patches of disorganization in the neocortex of children with autism. N Engl J Med 370: 1209–19.

17. Krishnan A, Zhan R, Yao V, Theesfeld CL, Wong AK, Tadych A, Volfovsky N, et al. (2016) Genome-wide prediction and functional characterization of the genetic basis of autism spectrum disorder. Nature Neuroscience 19: 1454–62.

18. Ozonoff S, Young GS, Carter A, Messinger D, Yirmiya N, Zwaigenbaum L, Bryson S, et al. (2011) Recurrence risk for autism spectrum disorders: A Baby Siblings Research Consortium study. Pediatrics 128(3): e488–95.

19. Glickman G, Harrison E, Dobkins K (2017) Vaccination rates among younger siblings of children with autism. N Engl J Med 377: 1099–101.

20. Sztainberg Y, Zoghbi HY (2016) Lessons learned from studying syndromic autism spectrum disorders. Nat Neurosci 19(11): 1408–17.

21. Landrigan PJ (2010) What causes autism? Exploring the environmental contribution. Current Opinion in Pediatrics 22: 219–25.

22. Mahic M, Mjaaland S, Bovelstad HM, Gunnes N, Susser E, Bresnahan M, . . . Lipkin WI (2017) Maternal immunoreactivity to herpes simplex virus 2 and risk of autism spectrum disorder in male offspring. mSphere 2: e00016–17.

23. Hornig M, Bresnahan MA, Che X, Schultz AF, Ukaigwe JE, Eddy ML, . . . Lipkin WI (2017) Prenatal fever and autism risk. Mol Psychiatry [Epub ahead of print].

24. Omer SB (2017) Maternal immunization. N Engl J Med 376(13): 1256–57.

25. Zerbo O, Qian Y, Yoshida C, Fireman BH, Klein NP, Croen LA (2017) Association between influenza infection and vaccination during pregnancy and risk of autism spectrum disorder. JAMA Pediatr 171(1): e163609.

26. https://www.ncbi.nlm.nih.gov/myncbi/janet.kern.1/comments.

Chapter 10. Struck by Lightning

1. Iqbal S, Barile JP, Thompson WW, DeStefano F (2013) Number of antigens in early childhood vaccines and neuropsychological outcomes at age 7–10 years. Pharmacoepidemiol Drug Saf 22(12): 1263–70.

2. Barile JP, Kuperminc GP, Weintraub ES, Mink JW, Thompson WW (2012) Thimerosal exposure in early life and neuropsychological outcomes 7–10 years later. J Pediatr Psychol 37(1): 106–18.

3. Turkeltaub JA, McCarty TR 3rd, Hotez PJ (2015) The intestinal protozoa: Emerging impact on global health and development. Curr Opin Gastroenterol 31(1): 38–44.

4. Donahue JG, Kieke BA, King JP, DeStefano F, Mascola MA, Irving SA, Cheetham TC, et al. (2017) Association of spontaneous abortion with receipt of inactivated influenza vaccine containing H1N1pdm09 in 2010–11 and 2011–12. Vaccine 35(40): 5314–22.

5. https://www.popsci.com/flu-vaccine-miscarriage.

6. Offit PA (2017) False alarm: The pregnancy vaccine scare that should never have been. Daily Beast, September 24. https://www.thedailybeast.com/the -pregnancy-vaccine-scare-that-should-have-never-been.

7. Eaton A, Lewis N, Fireman B, Hansen J, Baxter R, Gee J, Klein NP (2017) Birth outcomes following immunization of pregnant women with

pandemic H1N1 influenza vaccine 2009–2010. Vaccine, September 13. doi: 10.1016/j.vaccine.2017.08.080 [Epub ahead of print].

8. http://www.cnn.com/2017/06/21/health/vaccines-illness-european-court -bn/index.html.
9. Offit PA, Hackett CJ (2003) Addressing parents' concerns: Do vaccines cause allergic or autoimmune diseases? Pediatrics 111: 653–59.
10. Offit PA (2016) The HPV vaccine and autoimmunity: Reviewing the research (commentary). Medscape, September 15. http://www.medscape .com/viewarticle/868825.
11. https://vaers.hhs.gov/about.html.
12. CDC (1999) Withdrawal of rotavirus vaccine recommendation. MMWR Morbidity and Mortality Weekly Reports 48(43): 1007. https://www.cdc .gov/mmwr/preview/mmwrhtml/mm4843a5.htm.
13. https://www.hrsa.gov/vaccinecompensation/data/vicpmonthlyreport template5_1_17.pdf.
14. https://www.cdc.gov/vaccinesafety/ensuringsafety/monitoring/vaers/ index.html.
15. https://vaers.hhs.gov/faq.html.
16. https://www.fda.gov/biologicsbloodvaccines/safetyavailability/report aproblem/vaccineadverseevents/questionsaboutthevaccineadverseevent reportingsystemvaers/default.htm.
17. https://www.hrsa.gov/vaccinecompensation/vaccineinjurytable.pdf.
18. Wadman M (2017) Vaccines on trial. Science 356: 370–73.
19. https://www.hrsa.gov/vaccinecompensation.
20. http://news.nationalgeographic.com/news/2004/06/0623_040623_ lightningfacts.html.
21. Cook KM, Evans G (2011) The National Vaccine Injury Compensation Program. Pediatrics 127 (Suppl 1): S74.
22. https://www.cdc.gov/ncbddd/autism/data.html.

Chapter 12. "Science Tikkun"

1. http://video.foxnews.com/v/5405669524001/?#sp=show-clips.
2. http://www.nbcnews.com/id/8243264/ns/msnbc-morning_joe/t/coverup -cause-autism/#.WT3d4uvyvIU.
3. Kupferschmidt K (2017) The science of persuasion. Science 356: 366–69.
4. Rainie L, Funk C, Anderson M (2015) How scientists engage the public. http://www.pewinternet.org/2015/02/15/how-scientists-engage-public/ and

file:///C:/Users/hotez/Downloads/PI_PublicEngagementbyScientists_
021515%20(1).pdf.

5. http://www.researchamerica.org/polls-and-publications.

6. http://blog.chron.com/sciguy/2012/02/most-americans-dont-know
-where-research-is-done-or-who-funds-it.

7. Hotez PJ (2013) Forgotten people, forgotten diseases: The neglected tropical diseases and their global impact on health and development. ASM
Press.

8. Hotez PJ (2016) Blue marble health: An innovative plan to fight diseases of
the poor amid wealth. Johns Hopkins University Press.

9. Hall N (2014) The Kardashian index: A measure of discrepant social media
profile for scientists. Genome Biol 15(7): 424.

10. Hotez PJ (2017) How the anti-vaxxers are winning. New York Times,
February 8. https://www.nytimes.com/2017/02/08/opinion/how-the-anti
-vaxxers-are-winning.html?_r=0.

11. Hotez PJ (2017) "Science tikkun": Repairing the world through the science
of neglected diseases, science diplomacy, and public engagement. Scowcroft Paper no. 7. Scowcroft Institute of International Affairs, the Bush
School of Government & Public Service, Texas A&M University, January.
http://bush.tamu.edu/scowcroft/papers/hotez.

12. Gribbin J (2002) The first scientists. Chapter 3 in: The Scientists. Random
House, pp. 68–103.

13. https://www.aaas.org/program/science-technology-policy-fellowships.

14. Hotez PJ (2014) "Vaccine diplomacy": Historical perspectives and future
directions. PLOS Negl Trop Dis 8(6): e2808.

15. Hotez PJ (2015) Vaccine science diplomacy: Expanding capacity to prevent
emerging and neglected tropical diseases arising from Islamic State (IS)–
Held Territories. PLOS Negl Trop Dis 9(9): e0003852.

16. Hotez PJ (2017) Russian–United States vaccine science diplomacy: Preserving the legacy. PLOS Negl Trop Dis 11(5): e0005320.

Epilogue

1. Bruni F (2017) I'm O.K.—You're pure evil. New York Times, June 17.
https://www.nytimes.com/2017/06/17/opinion/sunday/im-ok-youre-pure
-evil.html?smid=tw-share&_r=0.

2. Hotez PJ (2016) Texas and its measles epidemics. PLOS Med 13(10):
e1002153. https://doi.org/10.1371/journal.pmed.1002153.

3. Hotez P (2017) The "Why vaccines don't cause autism" papers. PLOS Speaking of Medicine, January 20. http://blogs.plos.org/speakingof medicine/2017/01/20/the-why-vaccines-dont-cause-autism-papers.

4. Hotez P (2017) Autism spectrum disorder: If not vaccines, then what? From the Labs (blog), February 24. https://fromthelabs.bcm.edu/2017/02 /24/autism-spectrum-disorder-if-not-vaccines-then-what.

5. Moran MB (2015) Anti-vaxx websites, we're onto you. Time, February 11. http://time.com/4213054/anti-vaxx-websites.

6. https://www.bcm.edu/education/schools/national-school-of-tropical-medicine/public-policy.

7. https://www.cdc.gov/vaccinesafety/index.html.

8. http://www.who.int/features/qa/84/en.

9. https://www.aap.org/en-us/advocacy-and-policy/aap-health-initiatives/ immunization/Pages/vaccine-hesitant-parents.aspx.

10. GBD 2015 Mortality and Causes of Death Collaborators (2016) Global, regional, and national life expectancy, all-cause mortality, and cause-specific mortality for the 249 causes of death, 1980–2015: A systematic analysis for the Global Burden of Disease Study 2015. Lancet 388: 1459–544.

11. https://www.cdc.gov/nchs/nvss/deaths.htm and https://www.cdc.gov/ nchs/data/nvsr/nvsr65/nvsr65_04.pdf.

12. http://www.politifact.com/punditfact/statements/2015/feb/03/bob-sears/ what-cdc-statistics-say-about-vaccine-illnesses-in.

13. Smith TC (2017) Vaccine rejection and hesitancy: A review and call to action. Open Forum Infect Dis 4(3): ofx146.

14. Hotez PJ (2017) "Melanie's measles" is deadly and causes permanent neurologic impairment. Microbes Infect [Epub ahead of print].

Index

Note: Page numbers in *italic* indicate figures and tables.